Mental illness does not discriminate.

Unlike cancer and heart disease which can be encouraged by indulgences and excesses, illnesses such as schizophrenia, bi polar disorder, borderline personality disorder and many many others appear by magic and are thrust upon even the healthiest and fittest of souls. These illnesses are not uncommon, nor are they prevalent in any particular social group, yet they are little understood and still hold the stigma of shame and embarrassment. There isn't much sympathy for the man walking down the road naked and shouting obscenities to anyone who cares to listen. Nor is there much patience for the middle aged woman who tries to slash her wrists for the sixth time this year. Yet these people are everywhere and they are as ill as anyone awaiting chemotherapy or a heart bypass. We just don't want to confront them or acknowledge them. We fear them. How far have we really come since those vast, grey, Victorian sanatoriums?

I am a long term manic depressive. I have done things that can never be truly justified; things that are terrifying both to me and those who witnessed them. Whole lives have been affected by my 'crazy' actions. So how can such illnesses not be taken seriously?

I spend my life campaigning to bring mental illness into the focus of the general public; to try and shed a little light on what goes on in a 'broken mind' and to hopefully show people how it effects every aspect of a sufferer's life.

I offer no apologies for what many will feel to be very offensive and insensitive depictions in this novel. It is what it is....mental illness does not discriminate.

I am not mad....I am just unwell.

Joe Nunn

CROUCHING

In Random Places

BY

JOE NUNN

THIS BOOK IS DEDICATED TO JOANNE WILLIAMS
WHO I WROTE IT FOR WITHOUT EVEN KNOWING IT

AND TO MY SON WILLIAM, WHO I HAVE SPENT
TOO MANY DAYS APART FROM .

I LOVE YOU BOTH.

THE DAY BEFORE

Today's post to the CROUCHING in Random Places site:

In ham related news, the head of the CROUCHING community is pleased to announce that yesterday morning's picket of the Spar shop on North Hill went staggeringly well. As you know, I rarely travel outside into the city centre these days, but on this occasion I decided that the cause was worthy of the effort. I arrived at the said venue at ten past ten with my banner proclaiming, 'NO HAM WHAT A SHAM' held high above my head.

For those of you who have been on Mars for the last few weeks, yesterday's picket was the culmination in a long running battle I have been having with the Spar management, (although admittedly, they were completely unaware of this) in which I have encouraged a boycott of the shop. The boycott was imposed when it was brought to my attention by more than one of our student members, that on Wednesday 10th March, the shop ran out of all forms of ham. Obviously this was totally unacceptable and on the 13th March the boycott started. So far, I am pleased to announce that at least three people have since shopped elsewhere.

After picketing outside the shop for twenty minutes, a young woman manager approached me and after informing her of the reason behind the picket, she told me she was going to call the police. At last it seems someone is taking this ham related incident seriously. I celebrated this hard fought victory by CROUCHING outside Stratton – Creber Estate

Agents, performing a 110 degree left leg extension.

On a completely separate matter, I am receiving messages from concerned members regarding the measuring of their children's heads. I am working on a definitive size / age ratio and should have it sorted soon. In the meantime, keep measuring at least once per month and look out for any sharp growth patterns or melon like features. Never be afraid to stand behind your child and give their head a firm squeeze.

Kirkland Christie   Head of the CROUCHING Community

THE DAY BEFORE THAT

Post to the CROUCHING In Random Places site:

I have spent a wonderful couple of hours today climbing trees to a height of almost five feet. Yes, you read it correctly, five fucking feet! I never once thought I would ever achieve such heights, certainly not this year anyway. The view from one of the beech trees was remarkable from those sorts of altitude. I never realised that Thomson's are offering cruises to the Med for under £600 for example.

There will be those of you who worry about the Head of the CROUCHING Community taking such enormous risks, but danger is in my blood. I'm jumping off kerbs of over four inches in height later this week for Christ's sake.

Tomorrow's CROUCH will be held next to the car wash situated in the Shell petrol station on Plymouth Road, Plympton, at ten past ten. All members and non members are welcome but unfortunately the ban on Chinese remains in place and is unlikely to be lifted in the near future.

Kirkland Christie   Head of the CROUCHING Community

CHAPTER ONE

Not All Peacocks Have Feathers

CROUCHING Community Membership 2,859

The young manager of Peacocks, the clothes retailer, shook his head. He really didn't know what to do about me. It was bad enough for him all those months when it was just me, now he faced a dozen men and six women CROUCHING outside his store, in a small town, a suburb of Plymouth, at ten past ten on a weekday morning.

I was overjoyed at the turnout of the CROUCHING community. These were top drawer CROUCHERS. I always write CROUCH, CROUCHER, CROUCHING in capital letters. I don't know why; it's just the way it has always been and tradition was very important within the community. Well, it was to me anyway and I *was* the head of the CROUCHING community and had been for more than three years. I was in a particularly rewarding 140 degree double leg CROUCH. The March drizzle didn't bother me whatsoever and hadn't stopped the community coming out in force. I glanced across the other CROUCHERS and was pleased to see a good cross section of ages, from 20 to over 50, although most were in the 35 to 45 range, me included.

Mr Jones, the manager, who looked about 15 came out through the electric doors and stared at us disapprovingly for a few seconds. He turned directly toward me and said, "Mr Christie, this is the fifth time this month"

"I know. You must be thrilled," I replied without breaking my form even a fraction

"Don't you think the joke is wearing a bit thin?"

I kept my calm, even at such an offensive slur. I was used to this by now. "Mr Jones, as well you know, this is an official CROUCH. We are not on your property and therefore it is completely pointless moaning."

I scanned the other CROUCHERS and was pleased to see that none of them had broken rank or indeed had taken a blind bit of notice of the young Mr Jones. These were top drawer members. As usual many passers - by stopped to stare at us; a few gave me a thumbs up, one chap shouted out, "get on Christie you crazy bastard!"

People were used to seeing me CROUCHING on The Ridgeway, the principle shopping street in Plympton. For a long time it had just been me but in the last six or seven months, more and more people had decided to join me. The modern age of Facebook and Twitter had helped spread my CROUCHING gospel to the masses.

"You're all mad", snapped an angry looking elderly woman, whose spaniel was barking hysterically at Craney, who in turn barked back even louder.

"Thank you very much," I said politely, smiling at the woman. I rarely said anything whilst CROUCHING but I was in a particularly happy mood. I let her pass by and then looked at my watch. It said ten past ten. It generally did say ten past ten. In fact the battery had run out about twenty years ago and now everything in my world started and ended at ten past ten. I slowly stood upright and said, "I would like to thank you all for attending today's CROUCH outside Peacocks clothes shop on The Ridgeway. There will be a meeting of the CROUCHING community in the Sir Joshua Reynolds on Friday evening. I will lead a few practice CROUCHES at ten past ten. I hope to see you all there. As usual I would like to remind you all to keep measuring your children's heads on a regular basis." With that the CROUCH was over.

Farewells were said and there was a lot of handshaking and backslapping. I waved to Mr Jones who scowled at me before disappearing back into the shop. Craney and Dan, my two stalwarts of the community shouted some abuse at me and shot off up the road to their double parked transit. Lenny, who could always be relied upon to film a good CROUCH and single handedly had turned my crappy effort of a web site into something of real quality, wandered over and informed me about "some great camerage." He always said "camerage." I glanced uninterestedly for a few seconds at the footage he had shoved in front of me, before Nikki grabbed my arm to tell me she was off to Tesco. Nikki was one of my closest friends and along with Gemma was instrumental in keeping me out of the clutches of the men with white coats.

"Don't forget ham," I said. To be honest I said this to her and Gemma every time either of them went shopping. "Wafer thin," I added.

"Yes yes" Nikki said, already desperate to get away. I had demanded she attend this morning's CROUCH and she hadn't really wanted to come. She had said she had other things to do like cleaning her house and nonsense like that. She knew I'd never accept such an excuse. She scuttled off before I could issue more ham related demands. As I watched her, two girls came over to me. I recognised them as a couple of first time CROUCHERS who had been on the fringes of this morning's event and seemed to enjoy every second of it. I judged the pair to be a few years younger than me, about mid thirties, prime CROUCHING age and I vaguely recognised the shorter of the two, a freckly faced girl with blonde hair as a sometime regular at the Joshua Reynolds.

"Morning girls, did you enjoy the CROUCH?" I smiled warmly at the two of them.

They both laughed loudly and the one I vaguely recognised replied excitedly, "it was brilliant. You lot are all mental"

The other one added, "we saw you last week and just had to come along."

I smiled and introduced myself. "I'm Kirkland Christie, head of the CROUCHING community."

"We know who you are," they both said in unison, laughing loudly as they did so. The freckly faced one held out her hand and said, "I'm Dawn and this is Penny."

I shook their hands; Penny smiled sheepishly at me, her pale face going slightly pink as I stared somberly into her eyes. "The CROUCHING community welcomes all new members into its fold; except the Chinese of course."

"Of course" replied Penny looking unsure of what else to say.

Dawn took hold of my arm and said breezily, "do you fancy a coffee? We were just about to go in the cafe."

"Love to," I replied, allowing her to guide me across the road and into the small cafe that doubled as a florist.

A few seconds later we were seated in a corner of the busy little cafe, running the gauntlet of stares from the elderly clientele. They gave me concerned looks as I barked "good mornings" at them. The crazy guy who CROUCHED outside their windows was sat amongst them. I could almost taste their disgust. I soon forgot all about them and turned my attention to the two girls sat across from me.

"Do you want anything with your coffee Kirkland?" Penny asked as the waitress came over to take our order.

"Just coffee's fine," I replied. "I have a large ham eating session later on so best to save my appetite."

The girls looked at each, unsure as how to answer such a statement. After a short giggle Penny said, "ham eating session?"

I nodded, "Yep. Tesco's premium wafer thin."

Penny burst out laughing. A really loud laugh which caused another wave of horrified stares from a dozen pairs of elderly eyes. I looked at her impassively, not changing my expression whatsoever. "You think eating ham is funny?" I said evenly.

"It is when you call it a ham eating session." This from Dawn, who was also laughing, but at just under 100 decibels, unlike Penny.

"Ham is an extremely serious business", I went on. "In fact most of my important decisions tend to be ham related."

This time neither of them held back. They sounded like a pair of hungry seals. The waitress had brought our drinks over and looked decidedly uncomfortable as she placed the cups down on the table. I thanked her over the laughing and she quickly rushed off to a quieter table. I waited for the hysterics to subdue and said, "okay, putting ham to one side, how did you enjoy the CROUCH?"

"It was brilliant," replied Dawn. "You lot are so mad. I've seen you a couple of times up here and just had to join in. It's just so ridiculous."

"Where the hell did you come up with it?" Penny asked between sips from her cup.

"Outside Hall, Graves and Lee," I answered honestly.

"What?" Penny look puzzled.

"I was walking past Hall, Graves and Lee a few years ago when I suddenly had an overwhelming urge to CROUCH."

"Hall, Graves and Lee as in the car place?" Dawn was already beginning to crack up again.

"As in the *spiritual home* of CROUCHING." I waited for it. Sure enough huge roars of laughter filled the air.

"I fucking love it," screamed Penny oblivious to the disapproving glares.

"It was a life changing moment."

"Was it ham related?" asked Dawn almost spitting her coffee over me.

I thought about it for a moment before answering. "To be honest I don't think it was."

The two girls tried to get themselves together and when Dawn had finished wiping tears from her eyes she said, "I always see your rantings on Facebook. I thought this CROUCHING thing was about sex or something."

"A lot of people assume that. People have filthy minds in general. CROUCHING is exactly what it says it is. I just go out and CROUCH somewhere; anywhere, to be honest, hence the 'CROUCHING In Random Places' group. *Random* being the operative word."

"But if it's so random why are you always CROUCHING outside Peacocks?"

"Yeah, good point Dawn," added Penny. The pair looked at me expectantly.

"Because Peacocks is in need of regular CROUCHING activity."

This was too much for Penny, who bellowed, "CROUCHING activity?"

"Some places need a lot of CROUCHING outside them" I said attempting to justify my logic. "I have also been CROUCHING quite a bit next to the skip outside 44 Dudley Road. You know, get it done before it's removed."

Another explosion of laughter was followed by Dawn shouting, "sign us up!"

"Consider yourself members of The CROUCHING community. Remember to join the web site and Facebook group. It's the fastest growing knee bending related activity in the south of England."

"Priceless," laughed Penny. "You definitely cheer up a dull weekday morning Kirkland."

"Call me Kirk. I'm glad to be of service. The website will keep you abreast of the next CROUCH. I'm considering one for next week outside 'Barry's Half Price Bonanzas,' the cheap furniture place. It's crying out for a good CROUCH."

Penny drained the last of her coffee and wiped froth from her mouth with a serviette. She was an attractive looking girl when she smiled and she was smiling a lot. "What's with the dark glasses then? It's hardly bright sunshine out there." She nodded towards the window.

"One of the side effects of the medication I take is an aversion to bright light." This was actually true but there was an element of vanity thrown in too.

"What's the medication for? If you don't mind me asking?"

"I don't mind at all. Most of it's for ham related problems to be honest."

"I should have guessed," laughed Penny.

"And the rest is for various mental deficiencies."

"I should have guessed that to," Penny continued to laugh, just slightly less loudly than before. Loud enough to garner more withering stares though.

In fact I suffered from manic depression with a couple of personality disorders thrown in for good measure. It wasn't the best of mixes but I got by, in varying degrees of sanity, or quite often insanity and my illness had shaped the man I now was. Everything I did was in some way a reaction to my broken brain, whether I was jumping off kerbs or walking for endless hours with the sausage kings. My marriage had been ruined by my periodically manic escapades that had got ever more extreme. I had a young son to whom I was an embarrassment and I hadn't worked in more than three years. What little savings I had were rapidly disappearing and I was living on state benefits coupled with the ex wife's sofa and my friend Gemma's generosity. At 41 years of age life wasn't exactly 'starting'.

"So *how many* are there in the CROUCHING community?" Dawn asked, stressing the words, *how many.*

"There must be somewhere around 3000 by now I reckon," I replied matter of factly.

"3000?" Dawn exclaimed. "So how come there was only about twenty of us there today?"

"Eighteen actually," I corrected. "A huge turnout. Usually it's just me."

"Brilliant," laughed Dawn. "You are so funny Kirk."

"I take my CROUCHING very seriously. Soon the whole world will be CROUCHING in all sorts of random places. Do you know that in New York they had a CROUCH on Times Square last week? And not just a handful of CROUCHERS. There were almost 50. And they reckon they will have over 100 for the next one. The CROUCHING gospel continues to spread."

"You don't need to impress us Kirk, we're already sold," said Dawn.

I spent another twenty minutes or so, explaining the virtues and health benefits of a good CROUCH before getting up to head off for some awaiting kerbs. "Well, the head of the CROUCHING community must make his leave," I said somewhat dramatically, standing up from my chair. "I am off for a well earned bit of kerb jumping."

Penny looked up at me suitably impressed. "I presume it is how it sounds?"

I nodded. "Some of the kerbs are over four inches in height." I made a gesture with my hands.

Dawn again burst into fits of laughter. "You really are a fucking nutter Kirk."

I took that as a complement and left them to their laughter and headed off in search of some dangerously high kerbs to leap off.

It seemed strange to be walking without the sausage kings. That was what I called my two wire haired dachshunds. I say mine, but they live at the ex wife's house. I was quite well known around Plympton, not just because of the CROUCHING but also because of the sausage kings. They weren't your average sausage dog. These two had serious 'small man's' syndrome. As sweet as they may appear, with their bushy eyebrows, beards and big hairy paws, they liked nothing better than a good fight. Normally with each other. Not having them gave me the perfect opportunity for a bit of uninterrupted kerb jumping.

The walk to Kennel Hill, home of some infamous four and a half inch kerbs, was about half a mile and took me through the heart of the old part of Plympton, home to most of my extended family. I wondered if they would be proud to know that one of their very own was head of the fastest growing knee bending activity in the south of England. The town itself was the largest of Plymouth's suburbs, about five miles from the city centre. It was hemmed in by the river Plym estuary to the south and the towering sweeps of Dartmoor in the north. The town was predominantly residential with a smattering of small industrial estates and although working class, definitely at the higher end of the working class structure. Most of the homes were 1950's semi detached 2.4 children types, although there was the old part of St Maurice with its Norman castle and terraced streets. It had been my home for the last 41 years and recently I had found myself unable to travel even a mile outside of its borders.

I walked slowly along Underwood Road, a long narrow terraced street of cottages. My mother had been brought up here and it conjured up fond memories of an eccentric grandfather spouting off his own version of the gospels. Maybe a bit of him had found its way into me I thought, looking up at the old family home. I quickly pushed these memories aside and began to focus on the task ahead.

Numerous people asked me about kerb jumping. In fact most days I found myself having some form of discussion about it. This usually took the form of incredulous questions, with me justifying what a great past time it was. A very risky past time. Indeed, some of the kerbs were almost five inches in height. Unlike CROUCHING, which had recently become a group activity; sometimes anyway, kerb jumping was very much a solo pursuit.

I turned into Kennel Hill, admiring the old woods that stood high above the houses. I had spent many an hour running wild amongst the trees as a child; now those same trees looked down on me as I crossed the road and approached the highest of the kerbs. My heart began to beat faster as I admired how the kerbs dipped down to road level at the entrance of house driveways and then rose majestically above the tarmac to their highest peaks of four and a half inches. I stopped at what looked the highest of the kerbs and waited nervously as a car passed by. A couple of crows, sat on top one of those old wooden telegraph poles, squawked at me as if warning of the dangers ahead. I glanced at them briefly and then stepped up to the edge of the kerb. As I looked down I realised this bugger was getting close to five inches high. I counted down from three, held my breath and leapt into the air.

I landed about two feet out onto the road, a really good first effort. I hadn't considered how much easier it would be without the sausage kings in tow. Normally I would jump whilst holding their leashes and the pair of them would just stand rigidly on the pavement refusing to move; thus never allowing me the full thrill of the jump. Sometimes one of them would follow me into the road and the other would stay put, but it was never truly satisfactory. So being free of them I had a further half dozen jumps. When I finished I felt that it had definitely been one of my better kerb jumping sessions.

I strolled happily back the way I had come, beginning to feel peckish after the morning's activities. I decided to head to my parents house for a spot of free lunch. I checked my watch and saw that it was ten past ten; plenty of time. I was wondering which make of tomato soup mother would be serving up, when my mobile phone rang.

"Hello yes?" I answered in my standard abrupt style.

"Hello you." It was Lucy, the woman I was having an affair with even though I hadn't seen her in 25 years.

"Hey fat head. I've just been doing a spot of kerb jumping."

"You're such a twat." Twat was her usual term of endearment.

"Seriously. Kennel Hill. Great kerbage. By the way, you missed a good CROUCH this morning. You really need to get your arse in gear woman."

"I am going to come out. I promise."

"Friday," I replied quickly. "We'll be up the Joshua Reynolds for a bit of drinking and CROUCHING."

"I'll try," answered Lucy not sounding very convincing.

"Listen fat head, no more excuses." She had been putting it off for weeks.

"It's difficult for me Kirk, you know that."

No it's not. Jumping off of five inch kerbs is difficult."

"Twat," Lucy laughed. Are you online tonight? I need to chat."

"Chat now."

"I haven't got the time. In fact I have to go now. It's manic in here." Lucy worked in some sort of dull civil service job; land registry or something or other.

"What was the point of ringing now then?"

"To tell you to get online tonight. Right gotta go."

"Okay fat head, chat later." With that the call ended.

I stared at the screen for a few seconds as if expecting something to happen. It didn't. I put the phone back in my jacket pocket and went about considering the likelihood of Lucy finally coming out for a drink. Pretty slim I reckoned. Three times she had got close but each time had backed out with various excuses. Lucy was an old school mate that I hadn't seen since we both left 25 years before. I had reconnected with her through Facebook and although we had yet to meet in the flesh we chatted on line almost every night, sometimes for hours on end. It was quite obvious to both of us that there was a strong connection; she appeared to understand my problems and I was a good ear for hers. She was married with a couple of young kids and lived not too far from me. The marriage thing was a bit of a sticky area but to be honest I didn't really care. According to her Facebook photos she was a good looker, extremely so, but that doesn't always mean a great deal as anyone who has got involved with internet dating can testify to. Saying that, she was always attractive in school so there was every chance she still was. All I knew was that she's a very important part in my life and I was desperate to get her out for a night; although I was still worried about the potential for fat legs. I had a thing about fat legs especially in the ankle area.

Lunch at my parents was the usual affair; tomato soup, Co-op own brand; a reasonable choice. Staying with the usual subject thing, my mother told me off for not wearing a thicker jacket and told me of some illness that some cousin's nephew's neighbour's mate was suffering from. I left in plenty of time to get to my ex wife's house for my dog walking and babysitting duties. I say baby sitting in the loosest sense. My son was almost in his teens now and was definitely no baby anymore. The ex wife had been working nights for a year or so and from Monday to Thursday I would stay the night, crashing on the sofa until she returned the following morning. I would then push off for the day with the sausage kings. The rest of my week was spent at my friend Gemma's house. I had been there for about eighteen months and we had a terrific relationship. She was recently divorced and we had hit it off from the first time Nikki and introduced us. She had looked after me when my illness had been at its worse and I felt blessed to have her in my life. As for the ex wife, she tolerated me, which was incredible considering what a bad husband I had been. Our divorce had been finalised over two years ago but the marriage had been over long before that. I couldn't fault how well she brought up Zak, our son and she worked hard to ensure his life wasn't too adversely affected by our breakup and his father's shortcomings. Left to me his life would be a disaster.

It was mid afternoon when I knocked on the door. The ex wife had a rare day off but told me she would be starting her shift early today. I knocked again, loudly this time, knowing this would get the sausage kings going and sure enough I heard the ex wife screaming hysterically at them. This just made the dogs worse. Excellent, I thought. When she finally opened the door she said crossly, "why the hell did you bang so hard for?"

"Sorry," I lied and bent down to say hello to the sausage kings. Sunny immediately rolled over onto his back and started pissing in the air. The ex wife went mental and then Luca attacked him. Brilliant. There was all hell let loose. I managed to grab Luca by the collar and half strangling him, carried him through the house and flung him out the back door, into the small garden. Sunny had followed me and the pair of them stood growling at each other through the glass.

"You're such an idiot Kirk," the ex wife said, not for the first time, as she cleaned up the wet patch on the hallway carpet.

"What have I done? It wasn't me who pissed on the carpet."

"You know what I mean."

Somehow everything was my fault where the wife was concerned. She shouted at Sunny to stop growling and disappeared upstairs. I helped myself to a banana and put the kettle on. The dogs were still growling at each other by the time she left the house thirty minutes later. She left me with a list of chores and an order to ensure Zak was home by eight. Looking at the list I saw the first thing that needed my attention was to go to the shop and buy some juice and dog food. I was in need of a few beers for the evening so I decided to do this straight away. After five minutes of chasing Luca around the garden, I eventually managed to get both of the sausage kings on their leads and headed off on the short walk to the local Londis. It would prove to be one of the more eventful shopping trips.

CHAPTER TWO

SHORT ARMS LONG REACH

CROUCHING Community membership 2,903

There was still a slight drizzle in the air as I left the house with the sausage kings. They managed to piss on every lamppost and not just happy with that, each dog would go back to do another piss as soon as the other had finished. Without me yanking on the leads this would have gone on indefinitely. I wondered where all the piss came from considering how small they were. I had once seen them piss on the same post box over a dozen times each. On top of all the pissing they both liked to sniff each lamppost for as long as they could possibly get away with. Luca had been known to sniff the lamppost right outside the ex wife's house for nearly an hour and a half on one occasion. I suppose it's the same as me reading the local rag.

When I finally reached the shop I tied them up to the overflowing dustbin outside, which looked like it hadn't been emptied in months, if ever. The sausage kings were more than happy to have some free, piss sniffing time; the bin was obviously a sniffing hot spot. They quickly got feverishly to work with their noses.

Once inside I picked up a dozen Cobra beers, which were on special offer along with the juice and dog food. I decided that tripe was probably the one they'd least like, but they ate anything if I'm honest. At the counter I grabbed a couple of bars of Turkish Delight which I seemed to have become addicted to recently. I smiled at the attractive girl behind the counter as I handed her a £20 note, but she just looked through me and banged the change down on the counter, ignoring my outstretched hand. However, this little aside was nothing to what was waiting for me as I stepped out of the shop. In fact my heart nearly went through my chest. Patting the dogs on the head was a midget. The dogs were growling, as they knew how evil these little buggers were.

I stood motionless about ten feet away. Fortunately the midget wasn't one of those large headed ones. That would have really put the willies up me. I would have been forced to start shouting things at her. I steadied myself, took a deep breath and made my way over to the bin to untie the dogs, hoping that the midget didn't try and engage me in conversation. No such luck.

"They're such lovely little things."

"Yes," I replied trying not to look at the tiny figure bending over the dogs, who were eyeing her menacingly. "They'd be the perfect pets for someone like you."

She turned and looked up at me. "What's that supposed to mean?"

"Well you're undersized and so are they."

This didn't seem to go down well. She stood up to her full height, which admittedly was not very high at all and said angrily, "are you taking the piss?"

"I am merely stating a fact. They are not exactly Great Danes and you are somewhat short of normal height. Mind you, at least you haven't got one of those oversized heads like some of your lot."

Her face instantly turned a bright scarlet. "Who the fuck do you think you are?" She shouted at me.

"I am the head of the CROUCHING community actually," I replied.

"What?" I could almost see the steam rising from her. The sausage kings were getting agitated.

"The CROUCHING community welcomes midgets of the non large headed variety." I offered her my hand. I was being serious but she didn't appear to agree with my sentiments. She raised a small arm as if she was about to strike me and I shouted, "not the shins, anywhere but the shins!" She didn't strike me in the shins, but right in the nuts and it hurt like hell.

Just like every other man over the age of puberty would, I grunted in pain and felt my legs buckle under me. Tears came to my eyes and I slowly sunk to my knees. "I'm still taller than you," I managed to say through gritted teeth. Then the sausage kings decided to attack me. They did this whenever I had a play fight with Zak and now they were doing the same. Luca went for my genitals which, fortunately, were covered by my hands and Sunny just went about the business of randomly trying to bite me wherever he could. The midget walked away, but turned and gave me the middle finger (a fat one) and shouted something like, "fucking cock wanker" although I could have misheard due to the noise from the dogs. Thinking about it she might have said, "fucking pig, cock wanker," which I would have preferred.

It took me almost ten minutes to stand back up and to get the dogs under control. As I did so I noticed a bus had pulled up at the bus stop across the road. "Fucking dogs," I said and then looked across to see a dozen laughing faces looking at me from the bus windows. "Fucking midget fanciers!" I shouted as the bus pulled away.

Eventually I gathered myself together, untied the dogs and left the scene of my shame. Much to the pleasure of the sausage kings, I walked at a snail's pace, due to my aching man parts and they got loads of extra piss sniffing opportunities. As soon as I was back at the ex wife's I went in search of a bottle opener. I was in need of a beer. I searched through the various drawers and when I couldn't find one I almost decided to use Luca's teeth in revenge for the attack but eventually prised the top off with a knife. I filled a glass and took a long gulp of the cold lager. I squeezed half of the bottles into the crammed fridge, crushing a trifle in the process and as if by magic the sausage kings appeared below me, staring up at the hallowed glow of all their dreams. "You've got no chance boys," I said slamming the door shut.

I wandered into the lounge and sat down on the comfy sofa, which doubled as my uncomfortable bed. I resisted the urge to switch on the laptop, even though I was desperate to let the community know about my terrible experience at the hands of the midget. I never put it on until after Zak was in bed due to him complaining to his mother that I was always on it. I could do without another ear bashing from her. So I switched on the TV and watched the local news, drank my beer and slowly felt my nether regions return to normal. I was just about to open another bottle when my mobile buzzed. It would no doubt be a text from Zak asking if he could stay out longer. It was. I sent a message back of "NO" and knew that this would have the effect of shaving about three minutes off his extra half hour request.

I got up and went out to the kitchen to grab another beer and to feed the sausage kings, a task that always ended in violence. Sure enough today was no different. I filled two bowls at either end of the kitchen and watched as the dogs took about two seconds to demolish the tripe and biscuits. They then rushed to one another's bowl and licked them clean before meeting up in the middle for the usual scrap. I grabbed a bottle of disinfectant spray from under the sink and sprayed at them hoping to get them in the eyes. It did the trick and they disappeared off upstairs. My mobile buzzed again. "On my way" said the message. This meant he would leave the park in twenty minutes.

Zak finally arrived half an hour later, his face flushed and mud all over his tracksuit bottoms. "What time do you call this?" I asked as he bent down to greet the dogs who had reappeared from their hideout.

"Look at your watch," he said cheekily. I did. It said ten past ten.

"Do you want something to eat?" I asked knowing the answer was always yes, regardless of how much he'd eaten at his pals. He nodded and went upstairs for a shower. I put a couple of slices of bread into the toaster, the dogs watching my every move. When he came down in his dressing gown I passed him the plate with the toast on and he disappeared into the lounge to no doubt flop onto the sofa for an hour of TV. Within seconds he was shouting that the dogs were attacking him. Sure enough they were both taking random leaps towards the plate whilst Zak tried his best to shoe them away. I shouted the magic word "ham" and they shot into the kitchen and were sat looking up at the fridge before I had barely finished saying the word. I didn't give them any but it was enough to keep them away from Zak for twenty minutes. I went and sat down with him and asked about his day. It went something like this:

"How was school?"

"Crap."

"How come?"

"It just was."

"What did you do down the park?"

"Nothing."

"What have you got on in school tomorrow?"

"Shut up dad, I can't hear the telly."

And that was the extent of our conversation. I resigned myself to watching an episode of 'Family Guy' of which Zak had about 10,000 of on the Sky box recorder.

"Dad, you're like Peter Griffin," said Zak referring to the funny cartoon star of 'Family Guy'. "He's mental like you."

"Thanks mate."

"Well you are a *bit mental* aren't you?" Zak made the question sound like a statement. Of course he was right, I was a *bit mental*; perhaps more than a bit."

I sent him up to bed at just after ten shouting up to him to remember to check under his bed for midgets. He shouted back that I was a freak. "Love you to," I called up and got a grunt and heard the toilet door slam shut. I flicked on the laptop, marvelling at how long it took to get going. After ten minutes I was finally on the 'CROUCHING In Random Places' Facebook page. I used this to spread the CROUCHING gospel far and wide. I quickly glanced through the photos from the morning's CROUCH and was pleased to see some really good images. One had Mr Jones in the background; hand on hips, glaring at me. When I had finished with the photos I made the following post:

The head of the CROUCHING community would like to thank all of those members who attended this morning's CROUCH outside Peacocks on The Ridgeway, Plympton. I was particularly pleased to see a number of 120 degree left leg extensions undertaken. There will be a meeting of the community at the Sir Joshua Reynolds public house on Friday, with outside CROUCHES for all at ten past ten.

Kirkland Christie   Head of the CROUCHING Community

After I had made the post I spent a few minutes looking through some more photos which had been uploaded to the group page from various members around the world. I smiled as I looked at two youngsters CROUCHING on a car bonnet in Mexico City, half a dozen attractive girls CROUCHING in a queue for a nightclub in Barcelona and a number of brilliant ones from Molly in New York. There was CROUCHING activity in a number of American cities but New York was a real stronghold, mainly thanks to Molly and her student friends. The photos from her showed at least 50 of her students CROUCHING in Times Square to the bemusement of the many onlookers. I studied each picture carefully to ensure there were no Chinese faces amongst the CROUCHERS. I couldn't be sure the New Yorkers would be as discriminatory as me. I spent twenty minutes replying to messages and saying a few congratulatory words to Molly. When I had finished all my correspondence I made my second post of the evening:

Today I was subjected to a horrifying attack by a midget in what I can only describe as a vicious random assault. Fortunately the midget was not of the large headed variety or I don't know whether I would have survived, yet it does show the need to be vigilant at all times. These vertically challenged types are evil. I recommend measuring your children's heads on a weekly basis for the time being and always check under your beds before going to sleep.

Kirkland Christie   Head of the CROUCHING Community

It didn't take long for the comments to start popping up on the screen:

'Little Fuckers'

'Large headed freaks'

'Round the buggers up mate, it's the only way we can keep our children safe'

The last message had flicked on a light for me but before I could mull it over further Zak shouted from upstairs. "Dad, the dogs are doing my head in!"

I went upstairs and sure enough the sausage kings were jumping all over the bed, trying to find Zak who was hiding under the duvet. "Get them off me dad," he demanded.

I grabbed Luca and threw him out onto the landing. Sunny jumped off the bed and shot past me out of the bedroom and down the stairs. I could hear them growling at each other as Zak climbed out of his bed and barged past me on his way to the bathroom. When he came out I went after him only to find myself stood in a pool of piss. "For Christ's sake Zak, try and get it in the toilet for once. You've missed by six feet."

The sausage kings had come back upstairs and were already sniffing the piss, happily wagging their tails. As I unrolled a load of toilet paper to soak it up, Luca had begun to lick it up. I was half tempted to let him drink all of it, but I shooed the pair of them away and got down on my hands and knees to clean it up. I pulled off my sodden socks and threw them in the sink. I would have to borrow a pair of Zak's. As soon as I went back into his bedroom he said he was thirsty, holding an empty glass out for my benefit. I grabbed it, forgetting all about the socks and went back into the bathroom and filled it with cold water. When I handed the glass back to him he took the tiniest of sips and said, "this water's disgusting. It's toilet water."

"The water in the bathroom comes from exactly the same pipe as the water in the kitchen Zak." I explained, knowing it wouldn't be accepted.

"Dad, I'm gasping. I'm not drinking that, it's disgusting." He made a gasping noise.

I took the glass from him and walked to the top of the stairs and pretended to go down them. I waited for a minute and then went back into the bedroom and handed him back the glass. He took a sip and said, "that's better." I kissed him on the forehead and said goodnight, as he rolled over and closed his eyes. Half an hour later I was chatting online to Lucy. When I say chatting I actually mean live messaging. This was how the majority of our conversations took place.

"Hey"

'Hey fat head'

'You okay?'

'No. I've had a terrible midget related experience'

'So I see. Is that true what you posted?'

'Everything I post is true'

'Yeah right'

'Seriously. If I say I have been hiding in a bush making animal noises then that's exactly what I have been doing.'

'Twat. LOL xxx'

'I am considering organising a midget hunt'

'What are you like?'

'Hot and sexy'

'Hmm....'

'Are you coming out on Friday as promised?'

'We'll see'

'You have no choice now. You HAVE to come'

'Depends on the old man, he's being a bastard again at the moment'

'Y'

'You don't want to know'

'Is he buggering you?'

'Twat! Definitely not!'

'Are you buggering him?'

'TWAT!!! I saw the photos of you lot crouching. CROUCHING'

'Nearly. Did you admire my beautiful knee action?'

'It's just mad. You're all mad'

'Oi, I've told you before. CROUCHING is a very serious business'

'Well you never know I might be able to do a crouch with you on Friday'

'It's CROUCH!!! How many more times???'

'Sorry, CROUCH.'

'I shall wear my lucky red CROUCHING pants just in case you turn up'

'Lucky me! I want to come out but I'm really nervous'

'What about?'

'Meeting you'

'I quite understand. As head of the CROUCHING community I wield a lot of power. It's only natural for you to worry about being overcome'

'TWAT, you know what I mean'

'And don't go worrying that I might try to get you out the back. I've told you before, with all my meds I have no sex drive whatsoever'

'LOL. Off for a fag and a vodka top up. Back in a bit xxxx'

'K'

Our late night 'conversations' had been going on for months. Lucy had even told her husband that she was doing a course in work and that's why she needed to be on the computer so much. Apparently, in the Land Registry courses were all the rage. I gazed at her photo staring at me from the screen as I had done every night for more than six months. I had no idea when the picture was taken but whenever it was she looked really good.

Chestnut coloured hair, dropping just below the shoulders, a natural wave at the front, deep blue eyes emphasized by mascara and eye liner. A pouting mouth, the lips a ruby red and flawless skin, tanned but not unnaturally so. No hint of that orange sun bed look that so many women seemed to think looked attractive these days. Her large earrings looked expensive, as did the four rings I could see on her fingers. Fingers that were tastefully manicured. She obviously looked after herself and I was desperate to see her in the flesh.

I went into the kitchen and lay face down on the floor. I often did this but lately it was becoming more and more of a habit, especially when I was at Gemma's. Sunny had followed me in, no doubt hoping that the fridge would be my destination. He began to lick my face which I wouldn't have minded but his breath stank. After a couple of minutes I got up and opened the fridge. Luca appeared from nowhere and the two dogs looked up at me imploringly as I reached for a bottle of beer. I threw them a piece of ham each which they swallowed whole and then growled at each other. I went to the cupboard door under the stairs and this did the trick. Even the threat of opening the door to where the dreaded hoover was kept was enough to see them disappear upstairs. When they were puppies I had lifted them off the floor with suction and they never forgot. It had resulted in this great spin off and whenever I got fed up with them just the threat of the vacuum cleaner was enough to send them into hiding for hours. I considered going back to the kitchen floor but the beep from the laptop told me Lucy had finished her fag and refilled her glass.

'Hey'

'Hello fat head. Good fag?'

'Wonderful. What you doing?'

'I've been laying face down on the kitchen floor'

'Twat'

'I'm being serious. I am worried that I have a lino fetish'

'I really do worry about you'

'I worry about myself'

'I'm on my forth vodka. Bad day'

'You're an alcoholic'

'I think I might be. That's how shit my life is!'

'Well then, come out with me on Friday. Let your hair down. Be part of my crazy world'

'Fuck it I am coming out'

'You won't regret it fat head. You can even do a solo CROUCH'

'Don't even think about it or I won't turn up'

'OK I will protect you from all those nasty CROUCHERS. You will have to wear a very short skirt though.'

'And no knickers I suppose?'

'Good God! What sort of woman are you?'

'TWAT!!!!!!'

'I am so excited that you are coming out I am going to treat myself to a few slices of wafer thin ham and twenty minutes face down on the kitchen floor'

'What on earth am I letting myself in for?'

'Wafer thin if you're lucky'

'What?'

'It doesn't matter'

'Oh ham you mean?'

'I'll bring some up for you on Friday'

'I can't wait! You really know how to treat a lady'

'Don't worry, I won't forget. I never forget when ham is involved'

We prattled on for another half hour, me discussing the merits of ham and Lucy calling me a twat. Eventually she finally got to something important. I knew it was coming.

'Kirk, you know I am really nervous about meeting up with you. Our late night chats have kept me going over the last few months. You're really special to me'

'Don't worry fat head; I will be the perfect gentleman. It may surprise you to know that I too will be nervous'

'Really? Y?'

'In case you are not as hot as your photos'

'TWAT!!!!!!'

'I am serious. I have a reputation to protect.'

'Stop it'

'I'm sure you will be incredibly stunning'

'STOP IT'

'I've told the whole community that you're stunning'

'Do you want me to come or not?'

'Of course, just try and scrub up good'

'Right on that note I am off to bed. I will need as much beauty sleep as possible won't I?'

'Probably. And don't forget to measure your kid's heads before you do. It's the perfect opportunity whilst they are asleep'

'FUCK OFF YOU TWAT!!! XXXXXXX'

And on that note she was gone. On Friday I finally had my date, of sorts. She was married and I hadn't seen her in 25 years. I had been bugging Lucy to come out for weeks, I wondered what had changed her mind. I just really hoped she wasn't fat. Thinking about the fat situation I went back into the kitchen and once again lay face down on the kitchen floor. I had to consider a problem that I knew at some point I would have to face up to; two problems actually. The first was my lack of libido. I had had no sex drive whatsoever for the last three years due to the medication. I had been sex free, not even an erection. To be honest it was great having no sex drive. With no sexual urges whatsoever I was able to concentrate on the important things in life such as CROUCHING, kerb jumping and hiding in hedges etc. The other problem was one that had stuck with me since my last night of passion. I was going through the beginnings of the divorce and I began chatting to this girl I used to work with, on line again, and she had let me know quite openly that the next time I was in Exeter there was every possibility that a night of passion might be available. I had a work conference in Bristol coming up and let her know I would come and meet her on the way back to Plymouth. The problem arose when I was waiting for the conference to start and was mulling around in the reception of this place. I picked up a copy of an old FHM magazine and found myself reading the male problem page. In it was a letter from a guy who shouted "mercy mercy Uncle Percy" every time he climaxed. Now, for someone like me this was not the sort of thing I wanted to be reading right before a potential night of passion. Well, the inevitable happened and needless to say it didn't go down very well. I didn't just say it, I bellowed it out. I ended up sleeping in the car wondering what on earth she had against poor old Uncle Percy, whoever he was.

Now, I was here, laying face down on the kitchen floor worrying about such things. I would either fail to rise to the occasion or manage to, only to shout for Uncle Percy at the point of no return. It was a no win situation. Luca wandered into the kitchen and had a drink of water. I explained my problem to him but he just wagged his tail and stared at the fridge. I finally got up and realised I had yet to take my medication. It must have been all the midget excitement that made me forget. "Fucking midgets," I said to myself and threw a handful of pills into my mouth and washed them down with a gulp of lager. Anti – psychotics, mood stabilisers, anti – depressants, you name it I took it. I took the bottle of beer into the lounge and sat back down in front of the laptop to make a post on the CROUCHING In Random Places page:

There will be a CROUCH this morning at ten past ten outside the spiritual home of CROUCHING, Hall, Graves and Lee on Strode Road, Plympton. Strictly no Chinese.

Kirkland Christie   Head of the CROUCHING Community

Within minutes my nemesis Wendy Chang from the Yellow River Chinese Takeaway down the road came on line. I grabbed my beer, took a large swig and settled in for some late night fun.

'Christie you are fucking idiot' Brilliant

'Ah, good evening my yellow friend'

'Fuck you idiot'

'What is wrong tonight Wendy?'

'You that's what wrong. You pig prick idiot' Pretty good start.

'Is it because you are banned from CROUCHING?'

'I don't crouch. crouch fucking idiots.'

'It's CROUCH Wendy. Capital letters. Keep up.' I was prepared to ignore her English but not her wrong typing of the special word.

'Fuck you rassist pig'

'How am I racist?'

'You ban Chinese peeple crouching. Stupid pig fuck idiot'

This was great fun. I had another swig of beer.

'The reason I ban Chinese is due to small feet. It's a health and safety issue'

'Prik pig Health and safty issue. You pig prick health safety fucking issue'

'Due to small feet our yellow friends are prone to falling over when in the bended knee position'

'you are idiot rasits pig fuck'

'Don't blame me Wendy. Blame your parents. And by the way, your English is particularly poor tonight.'

'fuck off and di pig prik'

'Am I still banned from you take away?'

'you come in I fuck kill you'

With that final statement of intent she disconnected. I was thrilled by the exchange and immediately made the following post:

As the head of the CROUCHING community I often have to take decisions that people won't like or agree with. However, I feel I speak for the whole community when I state that under no circumstances will the Chinese be permitted to attend any CROUCH in the foreseeable future. This is not a racist decision but one made on the basis of health and safety. Small feet are not conducive to CROUCHING. Don't blame the messenger my yellow friends, blame your parents. And of course there is also the question of the sideways fannies. (That's front bottoms for our American friends – I know a fanny is a rear bottom over there)

Kirkland Christie   Head of the CROUCHING Community

I finished my beer and considered the sideways fanny question. It was something I had been worried about ever since a holiday fling with a Chinese bird in Majorca many years ago. My pals had insisted she would have a sideways fanny and burst into my room en mass just as I was about to get naked.

'You're too fucking early!' I had screamed at them and of course the moment was lost. I had managed a bit of a feel but to be honest it could have gone either way, no pun intended. Now it had become a bit of an obsession. In fact only the other day I had looked at a few oriental girls on line but they all seemed to have penises for some strange reason.

Just as I was about to switch the laptop off and hit the hay, Sammy Long Stockings came on line and messaged me.

'Hey CROUCHING man! I'm about to do my live show. Am I to be blessed with one of your strange requests tonight?'

Sammy was some strange middle aged woman from Boston, who basically liked to expose herself freely to anyone who could be bothered to go to her website. She was starting early tonight.

'Well Sammy, I was about to call it a night but seeing as you're a fellow CROUCHER I will look in on you shortly.'

'Great xxxx'

I went upstairs and looked in on Zak who was sleeping like an angel. I leant over and kissed him, then went to the bathroom, brushed my teeth, used the lavatory and stared at myself in the mirror. I wasn't sure I liked what I saw. I shook my head and went back downstairs yawning. The pills were beginning to kick in.

I clicked on Sammy's website and waited as the computer connected up with her live web cam show. After a brief wait her kitchen appeared and there was Sammy dressed in some sort of French maids get up along with a pair of marigolds. God knows what she was doing but I had an idea. I typed in: 'Hi Sammy, can you hold a carrot against your nose and say "where the fuck's Aunt Sally?"

I pulled a large furry throw from behind the sofa, at which point the sausage kings appeared and jumped up onto it. I made myself comfortable, stretching out, much to the annoyance of the dogs, who thought about growling at each other but instead flopped back down and closed their eyes. After a few minutes of watching Sally do things with a banana too rude to mention, she finally went to the fridge and appeared back in front of her camera with a large carrot. She climbed up onto the work surface and got onto all fours. Placing the carrot against her nose, she said, in what she thought was a sexy voice, "where the fuck is Aunt Sally".

I typed in, 'thanks Sammy x' and she shouted into the camera, "CROUCHER, you are one crazy cat" and blew me a kiss.

I turned off the computer and went to sleep.

CHAPTER THREE

THE SPIRITUAL HOME OF CROUCHING

CROUCHING Community Membership   3044

I was awoken by the ex wife just before seven. She placed a coffee down beside me and made a tutting noise as she picked up two empty beer bottles off of the coffee table. The sausage kings were going mad chasing each around the lounge before disappearing into the kitchen to stare at the fridge.

"I suppose you been up all night on that?" She said pointing at the laptop.

"Yeah, I've been looking at Chinese woman. Did you know they have sideways fannies?"

"Give it up Kirk. You don't half come out with some crap. How was Zak last night?"

"His usual cheery self."

"Right, I've got to get some sleep. I'll wake him up and get him in the bathroom. Do him some eggs for breakfast." She went into the kitchen and I followed her, needing a bit more milk in my coffee. She opened the fridge, much to the sausage kings delight and gave them a couple of mini sausages each. A bit like cannibalism I thought, but said nothing. "And don't forget to make sure he's got his football kit. Can you get here early tonight? I've got some overtime." She left me to go upstairs and I gave the dogs the rest of the milk, which they managed to drink without trying to kill each other.

By the time I had got Zak off to school and cleaned up the kitchen, it was well after nine. I had a quick wash, brushed my teeth and greased my hair back, for years now I had worn it in the style of a 1930's gangster. The dark glasses and thin gaunt face only added to the effect. I was in pretty good shape for my age, few grey hairs and still very little in the way of a middle age spread, although a few muscles on my thin body wouldn't have gone amiss. My once sparkling green eyes, now hidden away, had a bloodshot tinge and black lines underneath but still held a piercing look when needed. All in all I couldn't grumble at the hand fate had dealt me in the physical arena and I could hold myself up well to many of my younger contemparies. Even my modish dress style had a sort of retro chic which suited my 'out there' lifestyle. I wondered if I would be good enough for Lucy.

I left the house with the dogs and headed off in the direction of Hall, Graves and Lee. Already the urge to get there and CROUCH was building inside me. The sun was out and it was a glorious morning, the sausage kings were fairly bouncing along, clearly excited about going to the spiritual home of CROUCHING. We soon reached the scene of the previous night's midget assault, which again made me think about the potential of some sort of midget hunt. I was still mulling over the problem when I arrived outside the hallowed M.O.T. centre. Checking my watch I saw that I was dead on time; ten past ten. I stepped up onto the low wall in front of the garage, dragging the sausage kings up with me and slid down into a sublime 120 degree right leg slightly offset CROUCH. As I did so the dogs lay down on the wall just as they had a hundred times before.

"Get on Kirky boy! We thought you'd forgotten us this week," one of the mechanics shouted as he came out of the small front office to move a car. The workers all thought, rightly, that I was definitely not all there, and after a few months of regular CROUCHING activity had got used to seeing me and the sausage kings. In fact they would often offer me a cup of tea and a biscuit if the CROUCH coincided with their morning break. No such luck today.

"Are we too late to join your CROUCH?"

I turned around in surprise to see three young kids, students no doubt, rushing towards me along the pavement. Like me, the sausage kings were not used to having anyone else at a Hall, Graves and Lee CROUCH and they quickly made their displeasure known. Luca practically strangled himself as he leaped from the wall to confront them.

"You've started earlier than you said on the website," said the lad again in an almost accusatory manner. The two girls just behind were already bending down to pet the dogs who had quickly gone all soppy once they had realised one of them was eating a bagel or something. I recognised her from a CROUCH outside the entrance of the blind peoples home a couple of weeks ago. Nice arse but slightly goofy. I wondered if she'd been bullied at school. I resisted the urge to shout 'goofy' at her and looked at my watch.

"You put a start time of ten past ten," the lad went on.

"It *is* ten past ten," I answered, annoyed that I'd had to break my form to deal with the dogs who were now taking random snaps at the girl with the food. "CROUCHES outside Hall, Graves and Lee *always* commence at ten past ten."

"It's not even ten yet," he argued, looking at his mobile phone.

I tapped the glass of my watch and muttered something like "fucking Chinese watches," even though it was made in Japan. "In that case come up and join me," I added, "watch the sausage kings mind."

The three youngsters, none of whom looked out of their teens, eagerly stepped onto the wall and after a few seconds of awkward shuffling managed to get themselves into reasonable CROUCHES. The dogs settled back down and the four of us were left to CROUCH for a few minutes in peace before another of the workman came out and began shouting to his colleagues something about me grooming young kids. At this point the lad jumped down off the wall and began filming the remaining three of us. He was almost wetting himself in excitement.

"Is it some sort of porn film Kirk?" Someone shouted from inside the garage. I ignored all of this and remained focused on my CROUCH. I was well used to all sorts of interruptions. I let the kids enjoy being the first people other than me, Craney, Dan and Gemma to CROUCH outside the spiritual home of CROUCHING. I knew by what I had witnessed across the pond how quickly things could grow once the student population got involved. Let them have their moment, I thought. After another few minutes I stood upright and said, "thank you for attending today's CROUCH outside Hall, Graves and Lee on Strode Road in Plympton. The next CROUCH will be outside the Methodist church in Woodford at ten past ten on Sunday morning. And don't forget to measure your children's heads at least once a week." I doubted whether this was applicable to the three people with me but I said the words not wanting to disappoint them. Saying that, I often said it to just the sausage kings. With that, the morning's CROUCH was over. I nodded a curt goodbye, pulled on the dog's leads and walked quickly away, leaving the students bemused but happy.

I made my way to pick up my prescription, a weekly event that I found a drag but had managed over the months to make more tolerable by winding up the chemist, to the point that he had twice made me pick up my medication at a different dispensary. As I waited patiently for the sausage kings to go about their lamppost piss sniffing routine, I thought about the significance of the students turning up today. The word was definitely getting out about CROUCHING. It was well know amongst the community that I always CROUCHED outside Hall, Graves and Lee alone, except on very rare occasions. The fact that there were kids prepared to travel across town early on a weekday morning for a five minute knee bend, coupled with yesterday's unexpected turnout, was proof indeed that things were beginning to happen. I felt a wave of excitement run through me. At last people were starting to take notice of what I was offering. The years of solo CROUCHING was coming to an end. At the same time I considered the fact that Plymouth's students definitely needed to increase their drinking and drug taking. I wouldn't have dreamed of getting up at this ungodly hour when I was at university many moons ago.

I was dwelling on this and other more profound thoughts, such as whether to practice a bit of leaning against the wall of Rees youth club as I tied the sausage kings up outside the doctors surgery. For some reason they seemed content growling at a bicycle which was chained beside them. Entering the grey slab of a building, the collection point was just inside and to my absolute delight the woman with the wandering eye was working. I found her eye fascinating and would stand at various points many feet to the left or right of her when asking for my prescription. Today was no different. When I reached the front of the queue I immediately took three paces to my right before giving my name.

"Mr Christie isn't it?" The woman said turning her head slightly to look at me.

"Yes. Would you like me to stand somewhere more convenient?" I asked shuffling slightly to my left as I concentrated on which way her eye was going.

"Are you here for your repeat prescription?" The receptionist asked, her bad eye now looking somewhere between the top of my head and the ceiling.

"Aye," I replied, unable to help myself. She gave me a stern look, or shall I say half a stern look and disappeared to find my prescription. I stood at the counter trying to make myself go cross eyed in one eye but it was tougher to do than I imagined. By the time the receptionist returned with my paperwork I was pulling such extraordinary facial expressions the other people in the queue were giving me a wide berth. Thrusting out a hand, she passed me the piece of paper without saying a word, instead concentrating on the next person in line. As I took it I said to an old chap standing by the front doors, "you want to watch it mate, that woman behind the counter has got her eyes on you. Her right eye anyway." He gave me a startled look and I left him staring at the receptionist in confusion. I wondered if a proper persecution of people with wandering eyes may prove rewarding.

Next was the real fun part of the morning, the fat chemist. He despised me; in fact I think I was his most disliked customer and that included the entire methadone crowd, who always gave him plenty of verbal. The sausage kings wagged their tales as I untied them and then started fighting each other, which brought disapproving looks from a number of people as they went into the surgery. I thought about saying something witty but instead just yanked the dogs apart and dragged them down the path to the pharmacy, which was just a stone throw away. I walked straight in, ignoring the 'blind dogs only' sign and made my way to the counter.

"No dogs Mr Christie," said the fat chemist appearing from behind a stack of boxes.

"But it looks like rain," I replied making no attempt to do as he ordered.

"I'm sure they'll survive. You know the rules. If you want to collect your prescription tie them up outside."

"What if I don't want to collect my prescription?" I said evenly, still not moving.

"Outside Mr Christie, you know the rules," the fat chemist said, doing his best to be patient. He of all people knew the amount of strong medication I took, so understood I obviously had some bad mental problems. However, his patience only ever lasted a few minutes once he knew I was winding him up.

"One of them is blind. Your sign says blind dogs are allowed in." I smiled at him in what I hoped would be an angelic expression but probably just made me appear crazy.

"Out Mr Christie!" Obviously he was not in the mood to be patient with me today, so I turned on my heel and took the dogs back outside, tying them to the steps handrail. Unfortunately there was a golden retriever also tied up there and the sausage kings began to growl and snap, desperate to get at it. I made sure they couldn't, then went back inside only to hear the fat chemist shouting loudly, "how many times do I have to tell you Mr Jones? You need to fill in both sides. That's *both* sides."

I waited for him to finish his Basil Fawlty like customer service skills on poor old Mr Jones before handing him my prescription, muttering something about leeches under my breath, which the fat chemist chose to ignore. I sat down to wait on one of the four chairs provided and gazed at the tubs of expensive creams that apparently stopped you aging. After ten minutes the fat chemist shouted out my name even though he was stood practically beside me. Then he made a big deal of stating the fact that I didn't pay for my medication; that I was on benefits.

"Yeah, I'm too mental to work. All I'm good for is walking dogs. I'm not fortunate like you to have a fully working brain. Tell me fat chemist, would you look down your nose at me if I had a heart defect or a wandering eye?"

The fat chemist refused to rise to me and just handed me the large white bag. "Thank you Mr Christie," he said and turned his back on me. He was busy telling some other poor old bastard off for not doing joined up writing or something when I quickly rushed back to the counter and asked loudly, "tell me fat chemist, do you have one of those shoes for people with a club foot? You know, the ones with the big wedge soles?" I had been asking him this for months, for some reason I had become obsessed with getting one.

"Good day Mr Christie. Don't come back until your next prescription's due please."

I left him to his pill dispensing and went out to the sausage kings who had settled down now the retriever had gone. I walked them to Harewood House, a nice expanse of green where the local cricket team played during the summer months. I let them off their leads and sat down on a bench enjoying the feel of the spring sun as it poked out from behind one of the many clouds in the otherwise grey sky. Luca ran off to find me a stick to throw him and Sunny walked about three feet to do a bit of bin sniffing. No doubt that would be as far as he got, such was his love of piss sniffing. Luca came back with a piece of tree about four times bigger than him and then wouldn't let go of it when I went to throw it. I never knew why dogs did that. I was about to throw the log with him still attached to it when my mobile began ringing. I saw from the screen it was Nikki.

"Did you get the ham?" I asked without even saying hello. Nikki was used to this by now. In fact along with her pal Gemma, who she had introduced me to, Nikki was my best friend and I would have been lost without her; very lost indeed. We chatted about crap for a couple of minutes before she asked me if I wanted to go around to hers' later for a coffee. I said I would have to drop off the sausage kings; Nikki had four cats and the last time I unwisely took the dogs there it was like Pearl Harbour. With the arrangements made I hung up and immediately sent a text to Lucy demanding that she "ring me now woman." It was my standard demand when I was bored and sure enough a couple of minutes later she rang.

"Hello yes?"

"You wanted me?"

"I was bored."

"Charming. You really have all the chat up lines don't you?" Lucy laughed.

"Still on for tomorrow?" I asked, silently praying she hadn't changed her mind again.

"Yep. All cleared with the old man. It's about time he did his bit of staying in with the kids."

"Excellent," I said silently letting out my breath. "I will tell Gem to iron my best pants."

More laughter. "Twat"

"Don't forget, I am expecting you to wear your very shortest skirt and highest heels. I have promised the lads. Craney's even going to have a shave." Once again I found myself praying to God she didn't have fat legs.

"Don't Kirk. Or I won't come. I'm already nervous."

"How's everything at home?"

Lucy made a 'pah' sound which hurt my ear. "Fucking terrible. And I *mean* terrible."

"Never mind. I promise I will cheer you up tomorrow."

"You better. I need it. Right I've got to go. Some of us have work to. I will be online later."

"Okay fat head, laters."

I put the phone back in my jeans pocket and looked across the field to see the sausage kings both trying to hump a pug, whose owner was trying unsuccessfully to shoe them away. I walked over and asked the woman if her dog was on heat.

"He's a boy," she exclaimed as she flapped her arms at the chaos.

"Oh, sorry. It must be the sunshine making them frisky," I said matter of factly as Luca began to hump the side of Sonny's head. His 'pinkie' as I called it, appearing incongruously large for such a small dog. It reminded me I needed to see Craney about some Viagra. It was the old sexual problems that I worried about as I got the dogs under control and headed up to The Ridgeway to buy a pasty and a coffee.

I sat down on a circular bench outside my local, the Sir Joshua Reynolds, where I would finally meet Lucy the following evening. The dogs were in heaven as I kept managing to drop the insides of the pasty and in the end they must have had more of it than me. The inevitable fight started as they battled for the food. I let them get on with it, ignoring the worried looks from passing shoppers. Eventually, when it was apparent they meant business I threw them a big piece of crust each to shut them up. So much for my lunch.

"Fucking dogs," I said to the pair of them as they sat wagging their tales in expectation of further treats. I sipped the hot coffee and once more considered the sex problem. Was I just kidding myself that Lucy would be interested in me that way? Besides, she might be fat. Or smell. Yet I had the feeling she was going to be hot. The few photos of her on Facebook showed a pretty face but there was a complete lack of body information. There was nothing to prove or disprove fatness. Of late I had become increasingly intolerant of fat people even though I had plenty of fat friends. In fact the CROUCHING community was full of fat people. I think it was the fact that for nearly a year now and especially the last six months, Lucy and me had been in constant daily contact. We were intimate with each without being intimate, so to speak. We had an incredibly strong relationship without even meeting each other. Perhaps that's why it was so strong. Every day we shared our most private thoughts and concerns, I even told her about my urge to sniff a club foot big shoe. I needed her to be perfect. I had waited 25 years for her without even knowing it. And if she *was* perfect then I was in no doubt that our relationship would quickly turn to a sexual one. Or should I say wouldn't turn to a sexual one because of all my fucking problems. I consciously squeezed the bag of medication in my jacket pocket. What to do Christie, what to do?

I chatted to a few people who were passing by; one bloke, I think he was called Dave and was very fat, bent down to stroke the dogs and I thought he was going to have a heart attack trying to get back up. To make matters worse Luca tried to bite him which just sent his blood pressure soar even higher. I apologised and decided to head off to the ex wife's before anyone else decided to stop. I looked at my watch which said ten past ten and decided it was probably a little early to go back yet, so chose to take a long, roundabout route.

Although Plympton had been my home for 41 years, I had spent a lot of time working away. Many times during my working life it would have been sensible to move to the south-east but I had always resisted it. I had stayed firmly loyal to my roots. Work had entailed various sales jobs, a few successful, most not so and a stint in an optician's that was always going to end in farce. I went from travelling back and forth across the south of England clocking up thousands of miles each year, to now being practically unable to move further than a couple of miles in any direction, I was now absolutely glued to my roots. I no longer chose to drive and my refusal to leave Plympton caused me untold difficulties. Slowly but surely my life had begun to unravel as my illness took an ever tightening grip. My beautiful wife eventually could take no more and finally plucked up the courage to end our long relationship, keeping Zak by her side and leaving me to live my nomadic life. Without the steadying influence of a wife and home I soon became more and more wrapped up in my strange obsessions. It wasn't until Lucy came along that I began to finally see an end to the downward spiral.

I stopped walking to check out a couple of kerbs that appeared pretty high and I considered a few jumps, but decided against it at the last moment. I just wasn't quite feeling it. Plus the sausage kings didn't appear too keen. When it comes to kerb jumping you always have to keep safety in mind. Jumping off kerbs of over four inches in height takes total focus and it's just not worth the risk if you have any doubts. I thought about the ex wife again. She had no idea how ill I had become until she found me very close to death after an overdose. I had woken up one morning and decided on the spot that it would be a good day to die. I came around in hospital days later, my family in tears around the bed. Yet all I could say was how great it was to 'piss while I talk to you.' The thrill of having a catheter was much more important to me than being alive, or the fact that I had devastated my family. Really, from that point on my marriage was finished. Not because my wife wanted it to, but because I made it increasingly impossible for her. I chased women, drank too much, gambled too much, did everything too much. And when my moods went the other way I refused to leave the house or to speak to anyone for weeks on end. At one point I tried to chop my arm off in front of her, announcing how much I wanted to stay in. I was rewarded with an ambulance to the local A & E and a two week stay in the nuthouse. Whist I wandered around the locked ward ranting about Lord knows what, a woman turned up at my home to announce that she'd been screwing me. When I left the hospital I was only married on paper. Not long after that the divorce papers arrived and I signed them without regret or emotion. My now ex wife deserved a life.

A few months after the divorce I sank into a deep depression and barely moved for six months. Eventually I was given a diagnosis of manic depression or bi polar as they like to call it these days and was persuaded to take copious amounts of psychiatric drugs until the quacks found a mixture that seemed to help me. Well, they basically fucked my brain up until I am now only able to live this strange, repetitive, agoraphobic life in which for the last few years has only been broken up with the odd bout of depression. The CROUCHING had come to me out of the blue and now seemed to have totally taken over my daily life. I preached the benefits of it daily to anyone who would listen and spent hours each night hammering away at my laptop spreading my CROUCHING gospel and to me it was the most normal thing in the world.

You sheep go off to work or go on holiday or go for a drive in the country. Me? I am off for a fucking CROUCH. A 120 degree left leg extension.

CHAPTER FOUR

IT'S NOT MY HEAD THAT NEEDS FIXING, IT'S HER HEART

CROUCHING Community Membership   3104

I arrived at Nikki's mid afternoon. Fortunately the ex wife had been awake, as the sausage kings had raced upstairs before I could stop them jumping on her bed. I had been bracing myself for a bollocking and was relieved when it never came. I was told to be no more than a couple of hours and not to forget about Zak's English homework, no matter what he said.

Nikki was a couple of years younger than me and a beautiful girl. Her dazzling smile never failed to lift me and we had become great friends in the last few years. Along with her friend Gemma, she had helped me through many dark times and I loved her to bits.

"Hey Nikki," I said and kissed her on the cheek as she opened the door and ushered me inside."

"Hi Kirk. You okay?" She asked, cigarette in one hand, mobile phone in the other. All the women in my life smoked. Maybe that was the effect I had on them. "Coffee?" She added as I followed her through to the kitchen.

"Please," I replied, bending down to stroke one of her cats.

"So what have you been up to today?" Nikki asked me as she filled a kettle.

"Nothing too much. A CROUCH outside Hall, Graves and Lee which is always enjoyable. Guess what?" I asked and went on before she could say anything. "Three students turned up to join in. I told you, CROUCHING is at last getting the recognition it deserves." Nikki laughed as she looked for a pair of clean mugs amongst the clutter of dishes around the sink. I went on, "and I went to pick up my meds. The fat chemist was on. I tell you what; he is losing patience with me big time."

"You'll end up getting banned again if you're not careful."

"Yeah, that's what I'm hoping."

We sat in the conservatory with our drinks and talked about Nikki's kids and all three arrived home from school as we did. They interrupted Nikki's moan about some guy who had let her down and I had to wait for her to sort them out with some grub before I gave her my big news. "Lucy's finally coming up the Josh tomorrow evening."

"Really?" Nikki took an extra long puff on her cigarette at this information.

"Yep. Our 25 year enforced separation is finally coming to an end."

"Christ Kirk, I bet you're shitting it?"

I leaned forward in my chair. "I *am* Nikki. What if she's fat?"

Nikki laughed. "Do you want me and Gemma to come up in case you need rescuing?"

"It's a CROUCHING meeting. I expect you there anyway."

"Oh right. How could I forget?"

"And whilst I think of it, did you restock the ham yesterday as you promised?"

"Yes yes, I re-stocked the ham. Anyway, your Lucy's married isn't she?"

I nodded and replied slowly, "yeah but not happily."

"Just be careful."

"What, condoms, you mean?"

Nikki laughed and shook her head. "I didn't think you had it in you anymore. No, I meant that the last thing you need is to end up in the middle of some family drama."

I ignored this advice and stuck to the sex part. "I'm really worried Nikki. Have you got any Viagra?"

"Why on earth would I have any Viagra?" She answered lighting another cigarette. "Anyway, I wouldn't worry about that for the moment. Like you just said, you haven't seen her in 25 years. What if she's not your type?"

"But what if she is and she demands sex?"

Nikki burst into loud laughter. "Christ, I've never met a man hoping his date doesn't want to have sex with him."

"That's how bad my life is Nikki." I didn't even bother bringing up the whole issue of Uncle Percy and when I left an hour later I was even more concerned about the potential for disaster the following night. I made her promise to rescue me if Lucy's legs showed the least bit of chubbiness and headed back to the ex wife's leaving her shaking her head in a mixture of confusion, pity and laughter. I felt not in the least bit reassured after telling her my worries. If anything it just made me feel worse.

On entering the ex wife's house the sausage kings welcomed me as if they hadn't seen me in six months not two hours. Then, somewhat predictably broke out into violence much to the pleasure of Zak who came running out from the lounge shouting at them and generally winding them up further, if that was possible. The ex wife screamed at all of us, then kissed

Zak goodbye before shooting off, yelling over her shoulder a reminder about homework as the door slammed behind her.

"Do you want a coffee mate?" I asked Zak turning on the kettle and reaching for milk from the fridge. I noticed all my bottles of beer had disappeared.

"Yes please dad," he replied from the floor where he was rolling around with the dogs. This was bound to end in further violence, it always did.

"After you've had that we need to crack on with your homework. I'll give you a hand."

"Four sugars," he said, ignoring me.

I gave him two and took the mug into the lounge to where the play fight had now moved. Sure enough Luca attacked Sonny and a split second later the two dogs went hell for leather at each other. Zak jumped onto the sofa and started to throw cushions at them which just made matters worse and I had to bring the vacuum cleaner out of the cupboard and push it into the lounge, such was the intensity of the fight. Normally just opening the cupboard door was enough. Only a few times in the last year had I needed to actually switch the thing on.

"Turn it on dad," Zak shouted. "Suck Sunny up"

It would have been nice but once the sausage kings clocked the dreaded machine heading toward them, they instantly called a truce and darted up the stairs for the safety of a bed. They would probably squeeze under Zak's and stay there until they heard the fridge door open. Zak had been ready to film a 'hoover assault' on the dogs as he called it and was annoyed when they had finished their latest outbreak of dachshund on dachshund violence.

"Right mate, ten minutes and then homework," I said as I pushed the vacuum cleaner back to the kitchen. I was reading the local newspaper when he came in with his school bag half an hour later.

"Dad, Harry's mum told him she saw you in a bush up Harewood House last week making weird noises." Zak didn't or couldn't look at me as he said this.

"It was probably monkey noises mate." I replied matter of factly.

Zak still didn't look at me. "Are you really mental?"

"It depends how you define mental. I enjoy hiding in a bush and barking, just like you enjoy playing football down the park." Was that a good analogy?

"You're like a freak dad."

"I'm the head of the CROUCHING community son." This wasn't what Zak wanted to hear.

"Freak," he shouted and stormed out of the kitchen, leaving me standing alone thinking about which bush I had been seen in.

I left Zak to cool down and rummaged through his school bag, getting a handful of soggy sandwiches for my efforts. I ended up having to empty it completely and was rewarded with various food items which obviously dated back weeks. Eventually I found the homework in question and saw that it was to write an essay about someone he admired. I guessed he wouldn't be writing it about me. I wondered if he would ever be ready to take on the mantle of head of the CROUCHING community. He came back downstairs followed by the sausage kings twenty minutes later. His need for food outweighing any anger he might feel for me and after a 'feast' of pizza and beans, he finally put pen to paper.

"I'm not doing it about you, dad," came the expected response when I asked him who was to be the topic of his admiration. "It's going to be about Grandad."

I could understand this, as the ex father in law had proved a great support to Zak in recent years and always helped the ex wife when she needed it. "Good. Can I read it when you've finished it?" He nodded and started writing. This lasted about ten minutes before he started moaning that he didn't know what else to write and as usual I ended up dictating virtually the whole piece. I wasn't too bothered as the football was on and I wanted to watch it with

Zak, so as soon as he had dotted the last full stop I sent him upstairs for a shower. I had to bribe him with the promise of a small glass of beer in order to get him to tell me where his mother had hidden the remaining bottles. The next couple of hours went peacefully, the two of us sat on the sofa watching the box, but when the ex wife rang a few minutes after he had gone up to bed her timing was predictably impeccable. Zak was chasing the sausage kings around his bedroom with a fishing rod (I liked his style) as they barked wildly at each other. After an ear bashing down the telephone and the traditional toilet water saga, I was finally able to relax in front of the laptop once more. I say relax but you could hardly call it that. I had things on my mind as usual and they needed to come out.

I quickly scanned through the 'CROUCHING In Random Places' site and Facebook pages. The membership continued to grow and there had been at least twenty new photos uploaded from various parts of the world. I answered numerous messages and e mails, made a short 'tweet' about ham and then made the following post:

The head of the CROUCHING community would like to thank all of those who turned up at this morning's CROUCH outside Hall, Graves and Lee. It was a pleasant surprise to have some company as this has traditionally been very much a solo CROUCH venue. In future anyone wishing to attend a CROUCH at the spiritual home of CROUCHING are advised to turn up wearing false beards and John Lennon type spectacles.

Tomorrow's CROUCH outside the small shrubbery at 27 Moorland Road has been cancelled due to my continued attendance at the mental health department of Plympton Hospital. The meeting of the CROUCHING community at the Sir Joshua Reynolds Public House on The Ridgeway, Plympton is still going ahead tomorrow evening, with outdoor CROUCHING opportunities at ten past ten.

Kirkland Christie   Head of the CROUCHING Community

I carried on answering various messages from members and potential members for thirty minutes before making another post:

With Easter fast approaching I would like to remind members of the CROUCHING community that our group is inclusive of all religions and races. The exception to this is the Chinese of course. This goes without saying. On the subject of religion I hope all our Roman Catholic members will remember to bend their knees before the Virgin Mary on Easter Sunday. I will be making animal noises of a religious nature outside Woodford Methodist Church at ten past ten.

Kirkland Christie   Head of the CROUCHING Community

For some reason the thought of Easter had once more got me thinking about the midget problem. I was mulling it over as Lucy came on line and messaged me.

'Hey you'

'Hello fat head. You ok?'

'Not really. Third vodka already!'

'That bad?'

'Yep'

'Old man?'

'And bloody kids'

'Dog ok?'

'Twat. She's fine. The only one though. Yours?'

'In big trouble. Socks will be over their heads again if I have any more trouble from them tonight' I had gone through a period of pulling a black sock over their heads when they misbehaved and would enjoy watching them run into walls. Firm but fair.

'LOL. I'm nervous as hell about tomorrow night'

'Have some ham'

'TWAT! I'm being serious'

'A lot of people get nervous when they meet the Head of the CROUCHING community'

'Yeah right. I'm so honoured'

'You better believe it'

'Are you ever serious about anything?'

'Yes. Ham, CROUCHING, kerb jumping, hiding in hedges and badger impressions'

'TWATTTTTT!

'Fucking black and white bastards. Oh yeah, I forgot...I also like climbing trees to a height under five feet. Ash or rowans preferably.'

'You're so brave'

'I know. It's no wonder you want me'

'Want you?'

'Obviously you want me. If you buy me a beer I will let you touch me while I CROUCH, although not in the genital area of course.'

'Kirk you cheer me up. What would I do without you?'

'Smoke and drink more?'

'Probably'

Then just as I was about to reply Lucy messaged: 'Gotta go back later xxx' and with that Facebook kindly informed me that she was disconnected. I went and got another beer from the fridge, which was still not cold enough due to the ex wife's meddling and ignored the sausage kings who as always had appeared by magic the minute I went anywhere near the fridge. I took the beer back into the lounge, slumped onto the sofa and pondered on the midget problem. Something had to be done. After ten minutes of deep thought I turned my attention back to the laptop and made what I hoped would be a landmark post:

THE GOOD FRIDAY MIDGET HUNT

In eight days time the inaugural Good Friday midget hunt will take place. The aim will be to hunt down and restrain any midgets in your location especially those of the large head variety. I suggest storing them in your cellars or the boots of cars. You may even wish to dig midget pits in your gardens for the more aggressive types. I am well aware that this will be a risky and dangerous pursuit and no doubt a severe test of nerves, but we need to get to grips with the ever expanding midget problem. I will be at the Sir Joshua Reynolds Public House tomorrow evening if anyone fancies a pint and to chat over how we are going to put the brakes on these marauding little buggers.

Kirkland Christie   Head of the CROUCHING Community

As soon as I pushed the return key I went into the kitchen and lay face down on the floor. The sausage kings followed me in and both of them began to lick my face before the predictable growling started. "Give it a fucking break," I shouted, stood up and took a couple of steps towards the dreaded cupboard. They quickly vanished and I returned to the lino. "Fucking dogs" I said loudly followed by "fucking midgets."

As I closed my eyes and placed my right cheek against the cold floor, my thoughts once more turned to Lucy and the sex problem. It was a real dilemma. Mr Softy or Uncle Percy? Neither offered me any comfort. I decided the best thing I could do is to bring it up with my psychologist tomorrow and ask her to prescribe some Viagra. I could already imagine the fat chemist's horror as I demanded the blue pills. With this problem now resolved, at least for now anyway, I went back to the laptop. In the short space of time that had passed since I made the midget hunt announcement, forty people had already committed to the event. There were a number of messages relating to the subject:

'Yes let's sort out these little fuckers once and for all'

'Don't give them an inch Kirk, or should that be a millimetre'

'My sister's a midget but not of the large head variety. What should I do?

'What's wrong with midgets? They can't help the way they are born'

'You are one seriously sick twat'

'When you say about a large head, how large does it have to be?'

'Can I dig a pit in my neighbour's back garden to put them?'

'This is the best idea you've had since we spent the weekend stalking that bloke at the end of my street with the club foot'

The last message, from Craney, referred to the weekend a bloke with a club foot moved in down the end of his street and the two of us decided to follow him everywhere he went. I think the idea was to try and steal his big shoe but neither of us had the nerve. In the end we were resigned to shouting 'funny foot' at him from behind parked cars. Mind you, we were much younger and immature in those days; we were only 39 after all.

I re-read the other comments and made the necessary replies to those that needed one.

'I suggest you put a sack over her and put her in the boot of your car'

'The thing that is wrong with midgets is their height. And small arms'

'Yes, quite right. I am very sick indeed'

'Water melon like'

'When are you going to get me my big shoe Craney?'

For another hour I chatted online to various members of the community about the midget problem. Someone even gave me the address of a large headed one living less than a mile away. The news sent a shiver down my spine. I was still dwelling on it when Lucy finally came back on line.

'I'm back xxx'

'So I see'

'Child problem!'

'Have you been measuring her head like I told you to?'

'What is it with you and midgets?'

'They are evil.'

'Why?'

'What do you mean, why?'

'Why are they evil?'

'Haven't you seen the size of their heads for fucks sake?'

'You are such a twat. I really do worry about you'

'One day you will thank me'

'What would you say if one of *my* children was a midget?'

'I'd tell you to dig a midget pit in your garden for it, or failing that put it in a sack and stash it in your cellar.'

'LOL. You really are a twat'

'I take it from your ridiculous attitude you won't be attending the midget hunt then?'

'I think I'll pass. I am still trying to get my head around crouching'

'For fucks sake woman, it's CROUCHING!!!'

'SORRY. CROUCHING. So you were back on Strode Road today?'

'Absolutely. Hall, Graves and Lee is the spiritual home of CROUCHING'

'Why there?'

'No idea. I just stopped there one day. I think it was an epiphany'

'So is there going to be a lot of CROUCHERS at the pub tomorrow?'

'About fifty or so I expect'

'Really? I never know when you're winding me up'

'Yes really. And you best wear a low cut top so I can assess your first CROUCH'

'Piss off!'

'Gone south have they? It happens when you get to your age'

'Oi! There's nothing wrong with my babies'

'I've got the psychologist tomorrow'

'I saw something about that'

'She's fucking hopeless. She honestly believes she can save me from myself'

'I'd love to be a fly on the wall. What happens there?'

'She asks me lots of pointless questions and I give her lots of pointless answers'

'CBT?'

'More like MFI'

'Do you talk about CROUCHING?'

'Of course we do. What do you take me for? It's the single most important aspect of my life. I have tried to get her to sign up for it but she's like you'

'What do you mean by that?'

'She takes an armchair interest only'

'Well that will change tomorrow won't it? Surely you must talk about other stuff?'

'We do. Kerb jumping for one thing and the Chinese problem always comes up. If you're a good girl tomorrow I will take you to Kennel Hill for a few leaps.'

'Can't wait'

'It's life changing you know'

'Oh Kirk, you really do cheer me up'

'So you keep saying. Actually kerb jumping is a very serious business'

'TWAT TWAT TWAT'

'I don't mock your love of swimming'

'That's for keeping fit'

'And?'

'I want you to be serious for a minute'

'In the words of Doctor Fraser Crane, I'm listening'

'Who?'

'It doesn't matter. Go on...'

'I'm worried about you.'

'Why?'

'Your views are getting more extreme'

'You reckon?'

'Kirk, the other day you wanted to paint your bollocks with Tippex and climb on the roof of the Conservative Club'

'A very fine idea it was to. I still haven't given up on that one'

'But why? For what reason?'

'I don't recall but it would have been an important at the time'

'And all this badger stuff. Making badger noises at the Co-op butcher because you thought he didn't have enough ham on display'

'Surely you have to agree with me on that'

'Why do you get angry about it?'

'I was fucking outraged fat head. He even had the smoked stuff next to the fucking stilton.'

'See what I mean? I don't want you to get ill honey'

'I fucking will if that ham tastes of stilton'

'And all this badger stuff. Where the hell has that suddenly come from?'

'Black and white bastards. I've said it once and I will say it again'

'Kirk, sweetie, I worry about you constantly. I don't want you to be taken away by the men in the white coats'

'I'm fine fat head. You concentrate your worries on the midget problem'

'LOL, I give up! There is another thing though'

'Now what?'

'I may have something wrong with me. I had to see a specialist today'

'Fanny?'

'Twat. Wrong time to say twat LOL'

'What then?'

'I've got an irregular heartbeat apparently. I had a scan today and a load of blood taken'

'Why haven't you mentioned this before?'

'I really wasn't sure if anything was wrong until today. I'm still not sure. And besides, you have enough to worry about with all the CROUCHING and stuff'

'Oi! I am allowed to care about you fat head'

'I know xxxx'

'So what happens now?'

'I have to go back in a fortnight for more tests and another scan apparently'

'You'll be fine'

'Promise?'

'I promise x If all else fails I will transplant my ticker to you'

'I don't think I could handle your black heart'

'Blacker than the ace of spades'

'I'm really worried Kirk'

'Don't be fat head. The doctors know their stuff these days; other than psychiatrists and psychologists obviously.'

'Anyway, I intend to forget all about it tomorrow and have a large drink with all you nutters'

'You can let your hair down and be crazy for a few hours'

'I need it'

'That's my fat head'

'Just be gentle with me'

'Not a hope of that'

'What time shall I get there?'

'As early as possible. I'll be there by six. Or five even'

'Ha ha. I wish! I'll be there by 8.I will call you when I leave home. Right, I've got to go; his lordship will only wonder what I am up to'

'Stay for a bit'

'I can't. I'll see you tomorrow xxxxx'

'Ok fat head I promise you'll enjoy yourself xxxx'

'Nite nite xxx'

Once more I was left looking blankly at Lucy's photo on the screen, just as I had done for most of the last six months. I leant back on the sofa, yawned and thought about what I had just been told. Knowing my luck she would drop dead just as she walked into the pub. I dwelt on it for about five seconds and then went back to the business of midget hunting. According to my website there was now over 75 people already signed up for the Good Friday festivities and there was dozens of positive comments supporting the event. I knew the community would rise to the challenge, not that they'd have to rise very high. One message in particular caught my eye. It was from a chap in Bristol who said that his next door neighbour was a midget and this was just the sort of encouragement he needed to 'sort the short arsed bastard out once and for all.' Another message I turned my attention to was from a local community member called Julie who said she was only 4'9. Was she a midget in my eyes? I told her that as long as her head was in proportion with the rest of her body she was okay.

After an hour of this I decided to do a bit of online research into irregular heartbeats. Thirty minutes later I was none the wiser but worried enough to realise it could be serious. 'Fucking typical' I said to the sausage kings who were lying on top of each other on the armchair opposite me. Sunny lifted his head up to look at me and thought about getting up but gave up on the idea and flopped back down on Luca, licking his ears as he did so. This made me think about kissing. Now that I had decided that sex would be a disaster, I focused my worries on the simple kiss. I tried to remember the last time I had snogged someone. I can't recall snogging the ex wife in over ten years. You just didn't do that sort of thing when you had been married for a few years. Well we didn't anyway. I tried to remember a drunken kiss with a young sort out the back of the Josh on last New Year's. To be honest I don't even think we kissed. I think she licked my face a lot and then was sick over one of my shoes. I wondered if Lucy and her old man ever snogged. I went to the bathroom and reached for the tooth floss. It was complicated stuff all this dating lark, no wonder I stuck to CROUCHING.

After a couple of tweets, one about the fact that the only yellow people allowed at any CROUCH were typhoid sufferers, I grabbed the throw, switched off the laptop, waited for the dogs to settle and fell asleep.

'

CHAPTER FIVE

PSYCHOLOGICALLY SPEAKING I'M FUCKED

CROUCHING Community Membership 3,224

I arrived at the hospital for my session with the psychologist ten minutes before the appointed time although according to my watch I was a lot earlier. I wandered into the grey reception area; in fact the whole building was grey, one of those dull, square eyesores of 60's and 70's architecture. It was due to be knocked down in the next couple of years which would mean I would have to go to Plymouth's Derriford hospital about four miles away for my monthly 'therapy sessions.' This place was handy and was literally a stone throw from Kennel Hill and the glorious kerbs. I gave my name to the young receptionist and was told to take a seat. Apparently the doctor was running a few minutes late.

I ambled over to the far side of the large waiting room, sat down and looked around. There was only three other people beside me, one was a middle aged man who was staring straight ahead, not moving a muscle and the other two appeared to be mother and daughter. The young girl was stick thin, six stone if that and she huddled against the older woman as she caught my eye. I turned my attention back to the man and said breezily, "Morning. Are you here for the shrink?'

'Yes,' he said without moving; not even a twitch.

'What's wrong with you?' I was always intrigued by other people's problems.

'I have issues,' he said slowly and deliberately, still staring straight ahead.

'What kind of issues?'

'Issues of the mind.'

I nodded although he didn't see me do so. He appeared to be transfixed on a picture hanging from the wall opposite him. It was a print of a child with a small dog. 'I also have issues of the mind,' I said trying to engage with him further. For a couple of minutes he said nothing but all of a sudden he turned to face me, his droopy face breaking into a smile.

'I have membranes.' He slowly raised his hand and pressed a finger against his head.

'You get membranes?'

'Yeah, real bad ones.' He suddenly slapped himself in the forehead, hard enough to leave a bright red mark

'Oh, you mean migraines,' I laughed pointing to my own head.

'Sometime the membranes get so bad I can't see and then they take over my mind completely.' He slapped his forehead for a second time. 'You don't ever want membranes' he said looking at me fixedly.

"Fucking membranes," I said attempting to empathise with my fellow nutter, but he had turned back to face the wall and was once again concentrating on the picture. I sighed loudly and looked up at the ceiling. This was the world I inhabited. Fucking membranes. I stood up and began to pace back and forth; the skinny girl hugged her mother tighter and Mr Membrane continued to sit absolutely still, although his mouth was moving, saying some silent words to some silent world. I paced for twenty minutes before Doctor Johnson, or Diane as she liked me to call her, was ready to see me. "You keep an eye on those membranes,' I said to Mr Membrane as I walked past him; he didn't move an inch.

Diane was a good ten years younger than me although she dressed as if she was ten years older. Her mousy hair was pulled tightly back in a bun and coupled with her small round lens spectacles she looked more like a 1950's school mistress. Her face was so pale a year in the Med would not have been enough to give her a healthy complexion. She smiled and indicated at me to take a chair. "Now then Kirkland, how have you been since we last met?"

I leaned forward conspiratorially and stroked my unshaven chin. "Things have been going pretty well to be honest Diane. The CROUCHING community continues to increase rapidly and I have managed to find a further three roads with kerbs over four inches high."

She looked at me with an expression that gave nothing away. "So the obsessive actions are still happening?"

"I wouldn't call them obsessive Doc."

"How would you describe them then?"

"Satisfying."

She made a few notes on a small pad, stopped writing and thought for a moment, then asked me, "would you say these things give you pleasure?"

"Absolutely," I replied quickly. "I wouldn't do them otherwise would I?"

She made more notes. "Okay, what else have you been doing?"

"That's a very good question Diane," I replied trying to resist the urge to pick my nose. "I spent a bit of time last week tree climbing. You know the old rowan and ash combo. Not over five feet mind. That goes without saying of course. I noticed a nice ash outside the entrance here that has less than five feet potential. I might have a go at it after the weekend."

"Anything else?"

"Well I am still hiding in the odd hedge and making animal noises. The trouble is the noise tends to give away my location, which sort of defeats the object. As soon as I'm hidden the urge to bark or moo becomes unbearable."

I watched Diane write a few more illegible words onto her legal pad. "So tell me Kirkland, what exactly is the purpose?"

"To hide of course," I said incredulously. "Why else would I choose to be in a hedge?"

"Why indeed?" She looked at me over the top of her spectacles. "Who exactly are you hiding from Kirkland?"

"Oh all sorts. Old people, short people, Chinese, welders..."

The doctor raised a hand to let me know she got the idea. "Okay. What about your family. Have you been keeping in touch with your son?"

"Yeah we're good," I answered, "And the ex wife hasn't blown up at me for a while now."

She seemed to like this and scribbled some more stuff in the pad. I felt like saying 'big cunt flaps' to see if she would write it down.

"Does your ex wife or son ever ask about your health?"

"Not a lot. Only when they find me embarrassing." Like last night I thought.

"And do you feel like an embarrassment?"

"No, why would I?"

"Well most people would consider you hiding in a hedge embarrassing."

I made a dismissive gesture and said, "well they obviously haven't tried it have they?"

"And do you never get to the end of the day and look back at what you've done with your time as somewhat unusual?"

"If I thought it unusual I wouldn't do it would I?"

Diane sat back in her chair and thought for a few seconds. I looked past her through the window and could see my old school in the distance. We'd had numerous conversations about my schooldays and whether I was happy there etc. And each time I had said I was. It was as if there had to be some terrible event that had happened in my past thus causing the illness I subsequently developed. She nibbled on the end of her pen, almost nervously and said, "okay Kirkland, let's consider an action. Would you consider standing on top of a post box to be strange?"

"It's ridiculous," I replied quickly.

"What makes it so ridiculous?"

"What do you mean? Of course it's ridiculous." I leant back in my chair.

"But what is so different between standing on a post box and jumping off a kerb for example?"

I stared at her in astonishment. "I can see I am totally wasting my time here."

The doctor ignored my outburst and went on, "indulge me Kirk please. What makes the two different?"

I shook my head and looked at my doctor as if she was speaking Japanese. "Jumping off kerbs, and we're talking over four inches high here doc, is an incredibly dangerous but ultimately rewarding experience. Any old fool can climb up on a post box."

"But what makes one rewarding and one not?"

I let out a loud sigh and slumped even further back into my seat. "Doc we are going around in circles here. It's like comparing CROUCHING to shrugging." I crossed my arms letting her know that as far as I was concerned this exchange was over.

However, Diane was not about to let me off the hook so easily. "Let's try it from a different angle. How did you come to find that jumping off kerbs was a rewarding experience?"

"I woke up one morning with an urge to kerb jump. It's as simple as that."

"And was it the same with CROUCHING?"

"No, I was walking the sausage kings and had an almost religious like experience outside Hall, Graves and Lee."

"The spiritual home of CROUCHING?"

I laughed at the doctor's knowledge of my world. "Yep. In fact I CROUCHED there yesterday." I reached across and grabbed a cup of water from the dispenser while Diane scribbled away. I took a sip and waited for her to finish before I got onto the subject that had been troubling me ever since Lucy had agreed to go out with me. "I want to talk to you about a personal matter if I may Diane?"

"Of course Kirkland." She put down her pen and looked at me expectantly.

"As you know I haven't been in a relationship for a considerable time, certainly not of a sexual nature." Diane nodded but said nothing. I went on, "well I have a date this evening that I think may end up in sex."

There was a barely noticeable rising of Diane's eyebrows. "And you're anxious about this?"

I nodded. "Extremely anxious Doc. It's sending me to the kitchen floor again."

"Okay Kirkland. We know that when you end up on the kitchen floor it is related to anxiety so you are definitely right to want to talk to me about it. Do you know why the thought of intimacy is making you anxious?"

I loved the way she used the word intimacy as opposed to sex or a fuck. "Well I can't get it up for one thing. The pills see to that as you well know."

"It's a very common side effect."

"And don't get me wrong, it's been a great side affect. Having no sex drive whatsoever has allowed me to focus my efforts elsewhere."

"Such as CROUCHING I presume?" The doctor offered a rare smile.

"Exactly Diane. But now I have a hot date."

"Let's consider the event happening then Kirkland. How do you think you will react when, at some point, you are faced with the prospect of having sex?"

I shook my head and said forlornly, "I don't know. To be honest I will probably make my excuses, rush home and head straight for the lino."

Diane removed her tiny glasses and looked at them absently. I waited for her to say something but she didn't so I added, "you're a young woman Diane, how would you feel if some bloke you were dating rushed off to lay face down on the kitchen floor as opposed to jumping into your bed?"

"That's not pertinent here Kirkland. I'm sure it's not a pleasant dilemma you find yourself in but I can only really help you with the emotional aspect of your life, not the physical side. If you believe that the side effects of your medication are causing you serious problems then you will have to get in touch with your psychiatrist. Perhaps where I can help you is emotionally. Do you think you are ready for this sort of relationship?"

"To be honest with you I was hoping you would write me a prescription for Viagra. At least then I could give her one even if I don't enjoy it. If nothing else she'd get a shag out of it."

"The thing with sex Kirkland is that it is a very emotional commitment between two people." She looked at me in with what I guess she thought was an earnest expression. "Do you think it's wise to have sex when you are completely detached from the whole experience? Tell me, how long has the relationship been going on?"

"Well, I haven't actually seen her since 1985." I didn't miss a beat as I said this.

"1985?" Diane looked at me with a confused expression.

"Yeah. You could say it's a bit of a slow burner."

"Kirkland, where are you going with this? Our sessions are supposed to deal with your illness and how it affects your everyday life. Perhaps we ought to stick to this."

"But I'm telling you my illness is about to ruin this relationship because she's going to expect hardcore bedroom activity and I will be laying face down on the kitchen fucking floor." My words came out in an angry rant and I stood up as I said them.

Diane ignored my bad language. "Kirkland, let's be frank. If you haven't seen this lady for 25 years it can hardly be a relationship. I don't know what to call it but a relationship it probably isn't."

"It's a relationship via Facebook," I offered by way of explanation.

"I see." She gave me a look that said 'I might be patient but not infinitely so.'

"Do you Doc?" I said a little sarcastically.

"I will talk to your psychiatrist about those particular side effects for you. Is that okay?"

"Thanks," I mumbled, knowing my shrink would not change my medication whatsoever. I made a mental note to ring Craney about some Viagra as soon as I got out of the hospital.

Diane made a couple of entries on the computer, tapping noisily away at the keyboard which for some reason annoyed me immensely. Strange when I consider how much typing I did every night. Eventually she turned back to face me and said, "right then Kirkland, back to your moods. How have they been since our last session?"

"How do you mean?"

"Happy? Sad? Up? Down?"

"Well I know I have been extremely focused."

"Go on." The notepad was back out, the pen poised in anticipation.

"I have continued to concentrate on the Chinese problem and have also put together a plan which, if all goes well will see a shit load of midgets rounded up." The doctor raised her eyebrows slightly but not too much. She was used to hearing me make outrageous statements. I went on, "take the Chinese problem Diane. There is just too many of them. More and more takeaways are opening up, Judo clubs are everywhere, and even pug dogs are getting popular. Little by little the Chinese are taking over the world. It's only a matter of time. The newspapers are up in arms about Romanians coming over here but do any of them ever mention the Chinese? And what do they do when they get here? They fuck like rabbits because they aren't allowed to have sex in China."

Diane butted in, as much as to calm my rant as to disagree with my world view. "What you mean is that the Chinese Government encourages them to have only one child because the country was becoming so overcrowded."

"Exactly. They send them over here and say 'go to England and fuck like rabbits. Spread your yellow faces far and wide. Feed them chow mien and spring rolls. Teach them tai kwan do and say 'fank you please to everyone.' Before you know it we'll all be Chinese. It's inevitable. I check my eyes every morning to check for slitiness. Do you?" I stared at her pulling my eyes into slits. "I bet you don't. You just accept the inevitable. Well I never will. As long as my feet remain unbandaged I will walk the sausage kings a free man. My blood will never turn yellow!" I slammed my palm down on the desk.

Diane was scribbling away furiously as I made my regular 'yellow peril' rant. "I'm glad you're taking notes Doc. It's about time you started taking the Chinese problem seriously." She ignored me, put her pen down and turned to the keyboard again. She pushed a few buttons and looked up at me, her expression offering no reaction to my outburst.

"You mentioned midgets earlier. That's a new one."

She was right. I always spouted off about the Chinese at some point in our meetings but so far I hadn't raised my ever increasing midget concerns. "Listen Diane, I don't have to tell a woman of science how dangerous the large headed ones are."

"I'm sorry?"

"The *dwarfs*. The *large headed dwarfs*. A midget has a proportionately small body whereas a dwarf has a huge head; and small arms. Both are troublesome but it's the large headed ones that really freak me out. I was attacked by a midget on Wednesday and if it had been of the large headed variety I don't think I would have pulled through." I described the incident.

"Kirkland, what is it that scares you about midgets and dwarfs so much?"

I looked at the psychologist in astonishment. "Well for one thing they are short and for another, some have extremely large heads." I sat back and folded my arms. I knew my logic was irrefutable.

"Yes I understand that, but what is it about these physical features that upset you so much? If you saw a one legged man would that upset you?"

"Only if he was Chinese."

"Let's assume he's British."

"Then no, of course not. Why on earth would I be scared of a one legged man for Christ's sake?"

She persisted. "Well what's so different between the two?"

"Their height for one thing," I smiled.

Diane took a long deep breath. I was getting to her. "Forget the height. They both have disfigurements, an imperfect body."

I laughed loudly and said, "that's a bit harsh Doc. The poor bastard may have lost his leg in Afghanistan.

"Kirkland, you know what I'm driving at. What makes them so different? Would you treat a one legged man the same as you would a midget?"

"Of course not. What do you take me for?"

"I am trying to find the line you find acceptable when another is not. After all, a midget is just a small person, perfectly healthy, just the same as me and you."

"How fucking dare you compare me to a midget." I was stunned and shocked. "Does my head appear too big for my body to you?" I banged the top of my head.

Diane ignored my outburst and went on patiently and with a calm voice asked me, "I really want to get to grips on why you think midgets ought to be persecuted."

I leant forward placing both hands firmly down on the desk, took an exaggerated breath and replied, "of course they should be persecuted. I suppose you would have them running freely around the streets twenty four seven?

"Not quite the phrase I'd use but yes of course I do. Haven't you considered your views to be a bit strange? Extreme maybe?"

"I should have known you'd be a midget sympathiser. Maybe even a midget fancier." I took off my dark glasses and looked her straight in the eyes. "Tell me Diane; do you measure your children's heads each week?" She looked back blankly. "I knew it," I exclaimed loudly. "I just hope they never learn of this when they grow up. It's worse than smoking during pregnancy for God's sake."

The doctor put her note pad down on the desk slowly; up until then she had been scribbling away furiously in what looked suspiciously to me like Chinese. Their reach was everywhere I thought to myself. She waited for me to calm down before saying, "right Kirkland, I want to get to the very core of this. I want you to think long and hard about exactly what bothers you about midgets. And I want no mention of big heads or how short they are. I want you to think very hard before you answer."

I took about a second. "That's like asking to explain what a vicar does without mentioning Jesus or the church."

"Just try."

"They have fat fingers."

"I want no comments about their physicality."

"High voices?" I said hopefully.

"Try again."

"A worrying stare."

Diane shook her head. "What would you do if a midget walked through the door right now?"

I looked nervously over my shoulder. "Do you have any sacks or large bags? Between the two of us we should be able to bundle it outside. I could give my dad a ring and lock it in the boot of his car."

"Right," Diane said slowly, "and then what?"

"Well, I'm trying to locate a good place for a midget pit where they can all be kept. Failing that a cellar would be fine. Being so small they wouldn't need too much oxygen would they."

Diane held up a hand to say she had heard enough for the moment. "I'm finding your attitude quite worrying Kirkland."

"To lenient you mean? Don't worry, I've organised a midget hunt for Good Friday."

"Midget hunt?" Diane repeated.

"Don't sound so worried Doc," I laughed. "We won't be shooting the little buggers, just rounding them up. I'm considering digging a pit up Harewood House by the cricket pitch. The ground's still pretty soft this time of year. And get this, my mate brown Brian, the postie, reckons there's one living on the St Maurice council estate that has a head the size of a water melon." I emphasized this with my hands and said again excitedly, "a fucking water melon!"

"Take a breath Kirkland. Calm down. I'm growing increasingly concerned at what I am hearing today. As you know I like to use these sessions as an open platform for you to express yourself, but should I become concerned that you are posing a danger to yourself or others I have a duty of care to follow."

"You're worried about the midget stuff aren't you Doc?"

"Well yes, I'm extremely concerned."

"You're right to be concerned. Everyone should be. I mean, when you hear stories of water melon sized heads it sends a shiver down your spine."

"No Kirkland," the doctor said firmly. "I don't think you understand. I'm worried about your mental state. You are showing every sign that you are in the early stages of a manic mood episode. Your thought process is completely wrong. Are you taking your medication properly?"

"You know I have. I wouldn't be hassling you about Viagra otherwise."

She nodded and turned back to her computer. After thirty seconds or so she turned back and said, "am I right you last saw Doctor Brown at the beginning of last month?

I nodded. "Yeah, that sounds about right."

Turning back to the screen and typing as she spoke she said, "right, I'm booking you an urgent appointment with Doctor Brown on Monday and also I am arranging for the Home Prevention Team to visit you at home tomorrow morning. Shall we make it at your parent's house?"

"Yeah, I suppose." My normal mental health nurse came to my parent's home to see me every couple of weeks. The old man liked to keep abreast of what was going on in my strange world and mother just enjoyed anything to do with illness.

"Okay then. If you go back to the waiting room I will go and arrange everything."

Back in the now empty waiting room I stood staring out of the large window that gave panoramic views of Plympton. Again I gazed at my old school, wondering which classroom my son would be in. I tried to conjure up some 25 year old memories of Lucy but found it impossible. I practiced a bit of leaning, using an old looking radiator which felt like it might give way at any second. Just as I was getting into what felt like a pretty decent lean Diane appeared from one of the offices opposite me and I somewhat reluctantly ended the lean to walk over to her. She gestured for me to follow her back to the small office and I did so wondering what on earth the Home Prevention Team were all about. It sounded like something out of Nazi Germany. I sat back down in the uncomfortable chair and looked expectantly at Diane.

"Right Kirkland, I've booked you in to see Dr Jackson at ten thirty on Monday morning. Dr Brown is in London, but don't worry, Dr Jackson will have all your notes and I'll try and pop in as well. Also, the Home Prevention Team will call at your parents at eleven tomorrow morning. Now, I need to stress how important it is for you to be there. They will assess how you are and act as a direct link to your psychiatrist. If you fail to show there is every chance you could be sectioned under the mental health act. Do you understand Kirkland?" She waited for me to nod before going on, "I've written some phone numbers down for you in case you need to get hold of any of us." She handed me a couple of cards. "Someone is always available to talk to and to help you should you need it. And finally, I know you have your date tonight but I strongly advise you to avoid any alcohol for the time being, at least until Dr Jackson can asses you. It can have a real detrimental effect on your thought process and should you be heading into a manic mood it may hasten the condition.

"Spoilsport," I muttered quietly.

A few minutes later, after confirming that I understood all she had told me, I was back outside in what was left of the overcast morning. I rang the old man to tell him about the meeting and he predictably said how thrilled my mother would be. Normally she would put everything down to a thyroid problem. Malfunctions ranging from my own, to legionnaires disease would be summarily blamed on a misfiring thyroid. I wished that was all it was. That could be fixed.

I headed quickly away from the hospital, glad to be out in the fresh air after its stuffy atmosphere and midget sympathisers. I glanced at my watch to see if it was lunchtime. It said ten past ten. My stomach must be telling my lies.

CHAPTER SIX

25 YEARS? YOU HAVEN'T CHANGED A BIT

CROUCHING community membership 3,316

I was wandering aimlessly away from the hospital, half considering a bit of tree climbing when a once red Ford Fiesta pulled up alongside me. Calling it once red was slightly optimistic to be honest. It may have been any colour really such was the state it was in. The driver beeped a strangled sounding horn and I checked my stride and peered in through the passenger door window. It was crazy Terry, a stick thin, well spoken late fifty something alcoholic, extremely well known around the Plympton pubs. He was always good fun and a generous hearted drunk.

"Hop in Kirk my boy; I'm going up the George for a couple."

The trees would still be there tomorrow I thought so I climbed in, immediately becoming aware of the smell of stale alcohol and panicking to pull my seat belt on as we missed an oncoming van by about an inch.

"Bloody vans," said Terry rummaging under his seat and pulling out a half litre bottle of scotch. He used his teeth to twist the top off and took a large swig as he braked heavily for a junction. "Never travel without it," he offered by way of explanation handing me the bottle as he pulled out in front of a 'small' ten ton truck which was quite clearly invisible to him.

"You'd have to be fucking mad to drive around without a drink these days," he said in his posh voice grabbing the bottle back off me and taking another large swig. We somehow managed to reach the George Inn car park without dying and as I got out of the car Terry handed me a tenner. "Get the drinks in. Large scotch for me. I need a piss."

I left him to it and went through the back door and through the busy restaurant and into the bar. I said hello to a couple of familiar faces and ordered myself a bottle of Pils and Terry's large scotch. Five minutes later he strolled into the bar with a wide smile across his face.

"Hello Kirk, how the devil are you my boy?"

"Hello Terry," I shook his outstretched hand and realised he had no idea that he'd just driven me here. I passed him his scotch.

"That's jolly decent of you. A large one to boot. Good man." He took the glass then asked the bar maid to add a little ice. "I never drink the stuff straight up you know. Got to think of the old liver these days." He patted an area of his stomach where he assumed his liver was.

"Terry, you paid for the drinks," I said passing him his change. "You just drove me here." I laughed as he took the coins looking confused.

"Do I have the car?"

"Yes, it's out the back mate."

"How fantastic," Terry said rubbing his unshaven chin. "Fancy coming in town?"

"No you're all right Terry. I've got a hot date tonight."

"Ah, the old dating game." He tapped his nose a couple of times. "Online jobby is it?"

I nodded. "In a manner of speaking it is."

"You need to be careful with these blind dates Kirk. I went on one last year and she stank of piss. Pissy Paula I called her."

"I bet you still had a go though?" I replied smiling broadly. Terry always put a smile on my face.

"I had to Kirk. She had this huge mountain of a son who threatened to bop me over the nut if I didn't."

"Get away."

"Seriously; he was a right piece of work I tell you. He said his ma needed a good seeing to and that she'd bought a new dress and handbag. Drove me back to drink that did. Six months dry and between them they drove me straight back to the bottle. Sometimes when I close my eyes I can still smell her you know. Did you just say I had the car?"

"Yeah, it's out the back." I nodded in the general direction.

"Fancy going in town for a couple?"

I couldn't help grinning. "Love to Terry but I've got a date tonight, remember?"

He half nodded, looked around the bar frowning and then turned back to me. "Black bird is she?"

"No." I shook my head.

"Good job. The last black chick I had was in Derby, 1984. Miners strike going on or something? You remember, Arthur Scargill and his flying wotnots. Noisy buggers. Never seen so many police. Where was I?"

"Black chick," I said helping him out.

"Oh yes, tits like pillows. I asked her for a blow job and she threatened to stab me. Stank of piss."

We drank in silence for a few minutes, Terry lost in his thoughts of 1984 and the flying wotnots. I had picked up the local newspaper which was on the bar and was flicking through it without taking anything in. From behind it I asked, "have you ever fucked a midget Terry?"

"Yes, Dusseldorf in the late 70's, had a squint. I couldn't tell if she was in pain or not."

I folded the paper and put it back on the bar; looking at the black marks it had left on my hands. "Did she stink of piss?" I asked spitting on them.

Terry thought for a moment before exclaiming loudly, "come to think of it I'm sure she did."

I nodded in agreement with him and waited to see if he would offer any further insight to midget sex. He didn't and instead asked the bar maid to order him a taxi to go into town and asked me if I wanted to go with him for a few drinks. I shook my head and told him I had a date. "Chinese bird," I said to him.

Terry suddenly looked interested. "Good from behind. Tend not to wash down below though."

"And sideways fanny's to boot," I added seriously.

"Top waitresses though," said Terry draining his glass.

"Especially in Chinese restaurants," I said.

"Absolutely," barked Terry. "Right I'm off. Early night."

With that he shook my hand again and strolled resolutely through the bar and out of the exit. I stayed for another twenty minutes, finishing my beer and thinking about midgets smelling of piss. Just before I left there was a call for Terry that his taxi was waiting for him in the car park at the back. When I left he was still visible further up the hill scratching his head and looking lost. A truly great bloke I thought to myself and walked off in the opposite direction from him, making my way to Gemma's.

I stopped outside Peacocks as I could see Mr Jones fiddling around at one of the tills. I made a few monkey faces at him through the window and considered a quick CROUCH but decided against it. Why should he benefit for two CROUCHES in such quick succession? He gave me what he assumed was a hard stare but that just encouraged me and I ended up spending nearly ten minutes doing badger impressions in the doorway for him. As I walked past the Sir Joshua Reynolds or 'Josh' as we all called it I almost went in for a beer but decided against it. I needed to be fresh and at my best for my big date. I even resisted the urge to climb the horse chestnut tree hanging over the path running down through Harewood House, which had been enticing me for weeks. I did spend a couple of minutes checking out the softness of the grass though, thinking about the potential for digging a midget pit one night. I'd ask Craney to drop over some shovels so I was all prepared should the need arise.

When I reached Gemma's she was on the phone, glass of wine on the go as usual and a cigarette burning away in an over full ashtray. She smiled at me and motioned towards the fridge. I topped her glass up and poured on for myself. She was deep in conversation, talking about some 'dirty little slapper' but blew me a kiss as I took my glass through to the dining room where the computer was set up on a desk in the corner. Opening my Facebook page the first thing I saw was loads more people had committed to the midget hunt and a message from Lucy from very early that morning saying how nervous she was about her night out. She said she will have probably consumed half a bottle of vodka before she leaves the house. This last bit of news caused me to worry that if she was really drunk at the end of the night, she would be more likely to want sex. I cursed myself for not pushing Diane harder about the Viagra prescription. I brought up the 'CROUCHING In Random Places' site and quickly glanced through the most recent posts. The Americans had been busy overnight, uploading a dozen new photos from New York including a brilliant one of four girls CROUCHING on Brooklyn Bridge. I sent Molly and her gang a congratulatory message before making a few extremely random tweets about badgers and then made the post:

There will be a CROUCH outside Peacocks on The Ridgeway, Plympton at 1500 hours tomorrow afternoon. CROUCHERS are encouraged to make animal noises at the shop manager who today gave the head of the CROUCHING community a very dirty look. All members and non members are welcome. Strictly no Chinese.

Kirkland Christie   Head of the CROUCHING Community

"What is it with you and the Chinese mate?" I hadn't noticed Gemma come up behind me.

"Gem do we really need to go through all this again? Sideways fannies for one thing."

She laughed. "That was Nikki on the phone. We're having a few at hers before we go out. I've booked a cab for nine. I take it the big date is still on?"

I swivelled around to face her. She was four years my junior and looked not dissimilar to Nikki in that she too had brown shoulder length hair, tied back in a pony tail today, showing off a clear complexion and shiny green, blue eyes. I call them that but they were more green than blue. Just like Nikki she too was a lovely looking girl. "Yeah, so far so good. Mind you I could do with a couple of Viagra. You know how it is down below."

Gemma laughed loudly. She had a wonderfully loud laugh and used it a lot. "Yeah, I know, Mr fucking softy." Her northern accent just added to her charisma and she wouldn't have been the same Gemma if she didn't swear constantly in her Manchester brogue. "You better hope she doesn't fancy you."

"Marvellous ain't it? I finally meet a bird and I'm praying she doesn't try it on," I moaned to her.

"If you had told me about the Viagra I could have probably got you some but there's no chance now you silly bugger."

"Don't worry about it Gem. Anyway she might be fat."

"Oh right, because you're Mr fucking perfect aren't you?"

"I'm not that bad."

Gemma kissed me on the forehead. "You're beautiful," she said and disappeared back into the kitchen. I spent ten minutes staring blankly at the computer screen vaguely thinking about whether I was indeed beautiful before finally deciding that it was highly unlikely, got up and followed her. She topped up my glass and said, "if you want anything ironed bring it down now. I'm doing a couple of bits for myself." She held up a sparkly red top for my benefit.

"Very nice," I remarked.

"Well I thought I'd treat myself. It's the first time in four fucking weeks that he's had the girls. I'm going to make the most of it." She had six year old twins she adored and an ex husband she hated. I went upstairs and chose a pale blue Fred Perry polo shirt for the evening and it definitely needed an iron. I took it down to Gemma and we chatted about her week and the kids. Eventually she shooed me off to the bathroom saying that she needed me in and out in plenty of time for her to make herself reasonable.

I shaved and showered, taking time to wash my hair properly and to trim down below, just in case. After brushing my teeth and gargling with mouth wash I shouted down the stairs to Gemma that the bathroom was free and then remembered I hadn't washed all my pubes away and shot back into the bathroom to do so before Gemma saw them. She would have gone mental if I had forgotten. When I was satisfied the bath was spotless I went into my bedroom and rummaged around for my lucky red boxers; I've no idea why they were lucky but they were apparently. I pulled them on along with a pair of dark blue socks and used an inordinate amount of gel to ensure my hair stayed fully slicked back. I sprayed on some odourless deodorant and made up for this by applying a good splash of my favourite

Armani aftershave. Finally I took a look at myself in the mirror. Not too bad I thought but nothing a few months in the gym wouldn't harm. One day, I promised myself I will definitely grow some muscles. I sighed at the thought of it and pulled on a pair of jeans.

Gemma was just about to enter the bathroom as I wandered out on to the landing. "Someone smells nice," she said coming over to sniff me.

"Gem, do you fancy shaving my arse hairs?"

"Fuck off," she laughed.

"Seriously, I couldn't reach them in the shower." I gestured to a Bic razor in a pot next to the bath.

"Kirk, you've got as much chance as me shaving your arse as you shaving mine."

"Do you want me to?"

"Fuck off!" She rushed into the bathroom and slammed the door. "Ring up Nikki, she'll do it for you," she shouted as I heard the bath water running.

I thought about it but decided she was winding me up. I went downstairs and pulled on my polo shirt Gemma had expertly ironed, checked myself again in the mirror and went to the fridge. I rummaged around and finally found what I was after. I pulled two slices of the wafer thin ham from the packet and put them in my jeans pocket. I went back upstairs and banged loudly on the bathroom door.

"What now?" Emma shouted.

"I'm going to take some ham with me to give Lucy. Do you think two slices is enough?"

A few seconds later the door opened and Gemma appeared wrapped in a huge towel. "You're going to give her some fucking ham?"

"It's wafer thin. Sainsbury's Taste the Difference," I explained.

"Kirk you are fucking priceless," Gemma laughed shaking her head. "What's she going to do with some fucking ham?"

"Eat it of course."

"Listen, if any bloke gave me some wafer thin ham on our first date I'd fuck them senseless. Now can I please have my fucking bath?" She slammed the door in my face. "And don't go bringing any 'For Sale' signs home." She shouted.

"You know I can't promise that," I called back as I went back down the stairs. I grabbed a jacket, checked my wallet and left the house. I headed off to the pub for my big date. Strolling through the early evening streets I felt both nervous and excited, never a good combination for me. I knew this to be the case as I was soon looking at each garden hedge to see if it might be suitable for a bit of hiding. I tried to offset this urge by stopping at a couple of post boxes for short leans which, although took the edge off, still didn't entirely settle me. I fingered the cold ham slices in my jeans pocket, which had now made an unsightly damp patch. Should I give her one piece at a time or be bold and hand her both pieces? Would that appear a bit forward? In the end I decided to give her both at once. Show her what kind of man I was. 'Here's your fucking ham girl, how do you like that?' She'd be putty in my hands after that.

I stopped briefly at Mary Chang's Chinese Takeaway to see if she was working. The place was packed. I pushed my face up against the steamy window but there was no sign of her. Mind you, one of the three young girls, who I presumed were her daughters, did see me and she stuck a middle finger up at me. This cheered me no end. It was going to be a good night. As I walked past St Mary's Church the bells rang out for a quarter to seven. I checked my watch. It said ten past ten. I grunted and carried on walking, up through Harewood House where I again stopped for a few minutes to consider the digging of a midget pit. I really needed to focus on this midget problem now that the date of the hunt was set. Five minutes later I walked through the door to my second home, the Sir Joshua Reynolds Public House, or 'Josh' as us locals liked to call it. It had been my local since I was no more than sixteen and was a proper drinking pub, full of good solid working class men and women. It had the reputation, sometimes warranted for being a bit of a rough joint but it was my local and I always felt safe and welcome there, no matter what sort of crazy shit I had been involved in.

I walked into the bar which had about twenty people in it; the jukebox was blaring out an old 'Who' classic and a couple of my oldest pals were stood at the bar.

"Christie you CROUCHING cunt," boomed Carter in his usual soft manner. "A gay bottle of Holsten Pils I take it?"

"Please mate," I smiled and shook his large hand, then turned to Lenny who looked like he'd had a good few already. "You alright Lenny?" I asked him as he swiftly finished his pint ready for Carter to get the round in.

"Yes mate, I'm good. I take it there will be a spot of knee bending tonight?" He replied tapping his jacket which I took to mean he had his IPhone.

"I imagine there will be a little at some point," I replied smiling. "Probably about ten past tennish."

Lenny laughed, his always reddish complexion flushed further by an afternoon of ale. "I had a feeling it might be around that time."

Carter passed me my bottle of beer and the three of us caught up on each other's news. After ten minutes of this I announced that I had a date and when I told them who it was with they both looked suitably shocked and impressed in equal measure.

"Christ, I think the last time I saw her was about ten years ago," said Carter. "I think it was out at Endsliegh Garden Centre. Fucking place. Yeah, I remember because I smiled at her and she walked straight past me."

"Did she have fat legs?" I asked urgently.

"Fucked if I can remember. Anyway, I didn't know you were seeing her. And I thought she was married."

"Well no, I haven't been seeing her. In fact I haven't seen her since we left school and yes she is married."

My two friends laughed before Lenny said, "she was always quite tasty at school."

"That means fuck all now," Carter said quickly. "Look at my wife." We all burst out laughing again; Carter's filling the whole pub.

I dug into my pocket and reached for the ham. "Well I'm hoping she's still half decent. I've brought her up some ham. Sainsbury's Taste the Difference."

This time Carter's laugh drowned even the jukebox. "Stunning mate," he boomed, then added, "you're fucking spoiling her. I'd have given her Tesco's own brand on your first date."

"You'll make a rod for your own back," laughed Lenny.

"She'll want Marks and fucking Spencer's next time."

I held the ham in my open palm for them to admire only to see that it was covered in fluff. The pair of them burst out into ever louder laughter and Lenny said, "she will be putty in your hands mate."

"You can't fail with that Kirk," Carter said before changing the subject. "I see we're all off midget hunting? It's about time we stood up to those buggers." He stopped himself and said, "or should I say kneel down to those buggers?"

"I'm in," added Lenny. "I'm sick of seeing them all running wild in the streets. We should have done it years ago."

Carter nodded in agreement. "You're right about them running wild. I saw one playing football up at Lee Moor a few months back."

I nodded and we discussed the midget problem for a further twenty minutes as the pub began to fill with Friday revellers, many of whom I recognised as members of the

CROUCHING community. I nodded and said hello as they arrived and before long I was busy speaking to various people about tonight's CROUCHING opportunities and future CROUCHES. It was just before eight when I felt my phone buzz in my jacket pocket. I answered it knowing that it was Lucy. "Hello yes."

"Hey you. I'm a couple of minutes away. Can you come out and meet me?"

"Are you excited?" I asked, knowing that I certainly was now I'd heard her voice.

"I'm shitting myself," she replied. I could hear her puff on a cigarette.

"You should be. The pub is packed with people waiting to see you CROUCH."

"Don't! Now get outside," Lucy ordered.

"Okay," I hung up and walked outside. I leaned against the pub wall trying to look cool, but I kept patting the back of my head trying to ensure my hair wasn't sticking out. Then she appeared from around the corner and took my breath away. She was stunning. Really stunning. She broke out into a broad smile as soon as she saw me.

"Mr Kirkland Christie, how the devil are you?"

I gave her a hard stare and said coldly, "do I know you?"

"Twat," she said predictably and threw her arms around me. She smelt wonderful. "I can't believe I'm finally meeting you."

"You're not going to faint are you?" I asked as she finally released me from her grip.

"Shut up you twat and let me have a proper look at you. Take those bloody sunglasses off."

"They're my proper glasses. I can't see a thing without them," I complained as she pulled them off anyway.

"Now I can see the real Kirk. Wow, those green eyes. Christ, twenty five years."

I raised my hands as she tried to hand me back my glasses. "No keep them. You look half decent without them."

"You really are a fucking twat." She grabbed my arm and said, "now are you going to get me a drink or what? I am in need of a very large vodka and coke."

We went into the pub and made our way to the bar. I introduced her to Lenny and Carter, or rather reintroduced and left her in their hands as I ordered the drinks. As I waited to be served I leant on the bar and looked at Lucy. She was laughing away with Carter and Lenny, no doubt reminiscing about the old school days. She really was quite beautiful. Tiny. I had completely forgotten how small she used to be. If it wasn't for her high heels I would be seriously worried about her height and asking if I could measure her children's heads. She had dark brown hair pulled back over her forehead by a pair of expensive looking gold framed sunglasses. She was tanned, sun bed no doubt and her complexion was flawless. Her lips had a slight pout and were painted a shockingly bright red. Just the right amount of mascara enhanced her large, light blue eyes and as I watched her laugh she had the most perfect white teeth that I already knew were false; a present to herself when her grandmother died and left her a few quid apparently. She wore tight blue jeans; I'd been worrying about fat legs for nothing and her top half was just as good. Over a skin tight white vest, which showed her ample cleavage, she wore an expensive looking suede jacket. All in all she looked about three divisions higher than I would ever reach. And I was smitten.

I paid for the drinks and the second I passed Lucy her vodka big Andy grabbed me. Big Andy was Craney's housemate and a long term member of the community. The two of them lived in a drink and drug fuelled world that resembled Hunter S Thompson's 'Fear and Loathing in Las Vegas.' Big Andy allegedly ran a roofing business but that was open to debate. He placed a huge hand on my shoulder and said loudly, "evening Christie. My nephew's head looked a tad on the large size when I had tea over my sister's last night. What do you reckon?"

I shook my head at him slowly. "There's a lot of it about," I said sympathetically. "What I would do is stand behind him and squeeze his head as hard as you can for about thirty seconds at a steady pressure. You can shout things like 'be gone fat headed beast' at the same time for added effect."

Andy shook my hand. "Thanks mate. I've worried about it all night. Craney wanted us to go back and do a midnight raid. You know he's already started digging his midget pit in the back garden?"

"I had a feeling he would have." I answered smiling. I knew the midget hunt would be right up Craney's street. I caught Lucy's eye as Andy was talking and I could see her expression of slight amazement. Welcome to my world I thought.

"I'll have the transit up and running for the hunt; Craney's got hold of a couple of old sofas for the back, so we can carry plenty of hunters in comfort." Lenny and Carter both laughed at this but it was Lucy who commented first.

"I can't believe you lot are taking this midget thing seriously."

I gave her a stern look and removed my glasses to emphasise my disapproval. "Everyone should take the midget problem seriously, isn't that right Carter?"

Carter made an apologetic shrug. "What can I say Lucy? They are running wild. Something's got to be done."

Big Andy added a few choice expletives of his own before disappearing to the pool table, at which point more community members came in and made their way over to me. It was impossible to speak to Lucy on her own. I had an obligation as the head of the CROUCHING community and tonight was a CROUCHING meeting. As I was being asked about tomorrow's Peacocks CROUCH Nikki and Gemma appeared and grabbed Lucy like some long lost sister. Watching them instantly hit it off gave me immense pleasure.

"Oi Mr Christie," shouted Gemma, "have you given Lucy her present yet?"

"Shit," I replied, "I've forgotten all about it."

"Bloody typical man," laughed Nikki.

I pushed pass Lenny to Lucy and said, "sorry fat head, I forgot to give you your present." I pulled out the two pieces of ham which were now limp as well as fluffy and offered them to Lucy. Lenny almost spat out his lager. A bemused Lucy looked at the ham and then at me, obviously completely awestruck by my grand offer...

"Fat head, I've brought you this gift of two slices of wafer thin ham."

"It's Sainsbury's Taste the Difference," Carter shouted from behind me.

"You're so kind Kirk," Lucy said without making any effort to take the ham from me.

"You have to eat it," I said with a completely serious expression on my face. I meant it.

"It's all fluffy," Lucy whined, making a face.

"Its wafer fucking thin," I pointed out.

"I can't believe he's actually given it to her," I heard Gemma say from behind me.

Lucy took the ham from me and frowned. "It's a bit warm."

I nodded in agreement. "Yeah, sorry about that. It's been next to my arse for the last few hours."

"Well in that case I haven't got a choice have I? Give me your beer." Gemma reached across and snatched the bottle from me, put both pieces of ham in her mouth, took a long swig of the Pils and swallowed.

Gemma was ecstatic. "Kirk, you've met your perfect woman at last!" She shouted loudly.

I leant forward and whispered quietly in Gemma's ear as she took another gulp from the bottle, "I knew you had a ham fetish."

"Twat," came back the response as she finally finished with the beer. "Any more surprise gifts I ought to know of?" She said passing me back the bottle which was practically drained.

"If you're a good girl tonight I may show you how to hide in a hedge without being reported to the police."

Before Lucy could answer Craney appeared and grabbed me, his rough skinned hands a complete contrast to Lucy's. "CROUCHY CROUCHY time matey," he said loudly, waving an arm across my face which I supposed was meant to show me his watch but actually just displayed one of his 'homemade' tattoos; a strange version of the Holy Trinity of which two of the characters appeared to be ducks. I took a look at my own watch which said ten past ten, pulled Lucy close to me and said, "are you ready for your first CROUCH?"

"After eating that bloody warm ham I'm ready for anything."

I climbed up onto one of the tall bar stools which Craney immediately began to wobble; I aimed a kick at his head which appeared to do the trick and motioned for Gemma to get the barmaid to ring the 'last orders' bell a couple of times. After thirty seconds or so, the jukebox was turned off and on the third ring of the bell the bar fell reasonably quiet. Dozens of faces looked up at me in expectation. I raised my right hand slowly and said in what I hoped was a loud enough voice without shouting, "members of the CROUCHING community, I would like to announce tonight's CROUCH in the Sir Joshua Reynolds Public House on The Ridgeway, Plympton. This is a 120 degree left leg extension CROUCH and as we are holding up people's drinking will last for only sixty seconds. There will follow some photo opportunities outside at ten past ten. All midget hunting issues shall be discussed up here tomorrow lunchtime." I motioned for the bell to be rang again and jumped down off the stool to begin the CROUCH. As I did so, more than half of the pub's clientele followed suit. I held Lucy's hand as she endeavoured to get the best possible form for her first ever CROUCH. Most of the community kept a good silence although I did hear a number of pig noises coming from the pool table area which I presumed would be from

Craney and big Andy. There was some laughter and quite a bit of talking from the non members which always pissed me off but all in all the CROUCH was a sight to behold. After precisely sixty seconds the barmaid rang the bell for the final time and the short CROUCH ended to a loud cheer. Maybe fifty people straightened their legs and stood back upright, large smiles on their faces. Once again I had brought true happiness to their lives. Pub goers who didn't have the foggiest what was going on had joined in and no doubt would soon become converts. They ought to try doing it outside Hall, Graves and Lee in the driving rain on a January morning I instantly found myself thinking, not wanting to but being unable to stop the thoughts drift into my consciousness.

"That was amazing," shouted Lucy excitedly breaking me from my darkening thoughts as I stared at the fat legs of some young bird that I had never seen before but was acting like she was some sort of CROUCHING regular. "I can't believe so many people joined in." Lucy added.

I grinned at her, happy to be proving her doubts wrong. "I keep telling you fat head, CROUCHING is the fastest growing knee bending activity in the world."

"You're all mad. Shit, I need to do this more often," Lucy laughed.

"Well fat head, you can't say I haven't tried. I reckon I must have asked you to at least fifty CROUCHES."

"I know! I'm hopeless. Is it always like this?"

I thought for a couple of seconds and answered, "No sometimes it's a right leg extension."

"Twat. You know what I mean."

"It just keeps on growing. Everybody wants to CROUCH it seems."

As if to confirm my last statement I was dragged outside to the front of the pub for a load of CROUCHING photographs. Lucy joined Gemma and Nikki who were already outside smoking whilst I spent the next twenty minutes or so doing various CROUCHES with various people. I did manage to grab Lucy to do a couple with me which she performed admirably even with Gemma constantly shouting instructions of 'up a bit, down a bit' at her constantly.

When all the outside CROUCHING had finally finished and the community members were happy with all the photographs and videos which no doubt were already being uploaded onto Facebook and the constant bombardment of questions about the midget hunt had ended, me and Lucy were left alone together in the chilly late evening darkness. "Having fun?" I asked her.

"More than you can possibly imagine." Lucy replied offering up a gleaming white smile.

"CROUCHING, drinking, smoking, ham eating. It must feel like all your dreams have come true at once."

"Kirk you've no idea." Her smile was waning.

"Oi," I prodded her in the side. "Don't start going all wet on me fat head.

She smiled once more but I could see there was something troubling her. She sighed and lit another cigarette and said nothing until she had taken a long drag on it. She blew the smoke into the air above her and said softly, "I need to do this more often. Do you realise how long it's been since I've been out like this?"

I looked at her over the top of my dark glasses frowning, "listen to me fat head, you can come out with me and get drunk whenever you want to. I guarantee no two nights will be the same."

Lucy's eyes shone a bright blue that even in the poor light I could quite easily lose myself in. She was really something. "I wish," was all she offered in response.

"I mean it." I really did mean it.

She let out an even longer sigh and looked at her cigarette. "I know I could do with a break."

"Do you want to tell me about your dodgy heart?"

She reached out and squeezed my hand, her tiny fingers feeling cold. "Not tonight Kirk. I just want to forget all about that shit. Health, husband, home. The three H's." She burst out laughing.

I leant over and kissed her gently on the forehead. "Come on, let's go back inside and get drunk."

"I'm already drunk," Lucy giggled.

"Well let's get drunker. Is that a proper term? Drunker?" I said stopping in my tracks just as I was about to lead her back into the pub.

"Don't ask me. You obviously don't remember how thick I was in school."

"Actually I don't remember anything prior to February 10th 2007."

Lucy burst out laughing. "Don't tell me, your first CROUCH."

I gave her another poke, this time in the arm. "No. Last fuck actually. And it was truly awful."

Lucy squeezed my hand tightly. "You really are a strange one Mr Christie. Strange but incredibly refreshing." She reached up and kissed me on the lips. I noticed the complete lack of any sort of stirring in the groin region. The kiss was only a quick peck but it felt like she had crossed some sort of invisible barrier. As she gazed up at me I said, "Your lips taste of ham."

"Twat," came back the predictable response.

We went back into the noisy bar and spent the next ninety minutes drinking, laughing, dancing and hugging. When her mobile buzzed to inform her that her taxi was outside I couldn't believe that it was midnight. I walked her out to it, declining the offer of a lift home.

"I like to walk," was all I offered by way of explanation.

She kissed me quickly on the lips once more and smiling broadly said, "it's been a real blast. I have loved every minute." I just gave her a wink and watched as she climbed into the back of the taxi. As the car disappeared from sight I stood motionlessly, lost in my thoughts. She was everything and more than I had imagined. She was the one. I knew it before but now I really knew it. I could smell the faint aroma of her perfume on me and I actually felt a shiver run through my entire body. 'This is ridiculous' I said to myself and turned and looked back towards the pub. Through the window I could see Gemma and Nikki surrounded by about half a dozen men. I zipped my jacket and headed off into the night. Twenty minutes later I was lifting a wrought iron driveway gate off of its hinges to take back for Gemma. Thinking about it I could have got one much nearer to her house and saved an awful lot of effort but she was worth it. I threw it into her small front garden next to the 'For Sale' signs and went indoors. When Gemma crashed in about an hour later, roaring drunk, she said it was the nicest present anyone had ever given her.

"She's fucking beautiful mate," Gemma slurred ten minutes later as we sat on the kitchen stools drinking coffee.

"I know Gem. She's such a nice girl too."

"I still can't believe she ate that fucking ham. She's obviously besotted poor cow."

"I'm glad you like her," I went on, anxious to hear Gemma's viewpoint on all things Lucy. "She was a bit nervous about meeting you and Nikki."

"Nervous about meeting me and Nik?" Gemma broke into one of her trademark loud laughs. "Fucking hell mate, I can't see how she can be nervous about anyone after meeting you. She's obviously half mad herself."

"Yeah alright," I said impatiently. "She just realises what she's been missing all these years. Twenty five years of loss."

"You don't half come out with some fucking rubbish Kirk," Gemma said still laughing. "And long may it last," she added before falling off her stool, at which point, after a long stream of expletives she announced she was off to bed. "Do not wake me at some ungodly hour to tell me about fresh fish seen off the coast of France or whatever crap it was last time, or I will do what the midget did to you only much, much, worse."

"Ok Gem, sweet dreams." I said sweetly.

"I'll probably dream off melon fucking heads or whatever it is you keep going on about."

"Don't forget to check under your bed before you turn the light off."

"Fuck off!" And with that I was left alone in the kitchen.

I finished my coffee, listening intently to Gemma clattering around above me. Finally after a loud crash and a loud 'oh fuck it' the house fell totally silent. I remembered I had yet to take my pills and used this excuse to boil the kettle again for another coffee rather than just have a glass of water. I wasn't quite ready to hit the hay yet. Things needed to be said on the computer, which Gemma had kindly forgotten to switch off before she had gone out. The first thing I did was send a private message to Lucy:

'Hi fat head, I just wanted to say how great it was to finally see you once again in the flesh. Obviously I was very disappointed that you looked years older than your forty years and you smelt like you hadn't seen a bar of soap in a week, but you did eat the ham and in my eyes that goes some way in making up for your many other deficiencies. I look forward to feeding you more food items in the near future.'

I chuckled as I reread it and after making myself a third coffee I brought up onto the screen the 'CROUCHING in Random Places' site. Just as I had hoped there was already nearly fifty new photos uploaded from the earlier CROUCHING activities and exactly ten included the image of Lucy. I clicked back and forth between each one, scrutinising every possible detail over and over. Again I found myself thinking how stunning she was. I couldn't wait to see her once more in the flesh and this time I would ensure it was only a matter of days not years. I must have stared at the images of her for well over an hour, so lost was I in her beauty.

To round off a perfect evening, when I checked my messages relating to the midget hunt there was over twenty from midgets and midget sympathisers (even midget fanciers I dare say) calling me every name under the sun. One midget (non large head variety) from Budapest of all places, had sent a photo of himself brandishing a huge meat cleaver with the words 'I will chop off your balls if you have any that is" written as an attached message. Brilliant, I thought. Things were moving along nicely. I retired to my bed a contented man.

CHAPTER SEVEN

ANIMAL CRACKERS

CROUCHING Community Membership 3,512

Saturday began with a headache, a severe dizziness due to taking my pills so late and a text from the ex wife summoning me to her house that morning. Cursing, I sent a message back saying I had to see my mental health people at eleven thirty but she replied insisting that it was important that she saw me and that she would drop me over to my parents house in time for my appointment. I crawled out of bed and made my way to the bathroom and a shower. The Doc was right about mixing too much booze with the pills. It was about the only thing she had ever got correct in all the time I had been seeing her. I turned the shower to cold trying to sort out just how correct she was. The cold water did help slightly as I tried not to swear at the chill of the icy needles of water, for fear of waking Gemma and all the problems that would lead to. Eventually, after a long session of aggressive teeth brushing and half a gallon of black coffee; I was definitely an addict, I headed off to the ex wife's arriving just on ten past ten.

"Dad's paid for all of us to fly out to see my uncle," The ex wife said to me as I crunched on a piece of toast and jam; the sausage kings staring up at me expectantly, while at the same time somehow manage to growl at each other.

"That's good of him." The ex wife's uncle Dave, her father's younger brother lived in Italy. "When?"

"Monday. For two weeks."

I swore under my breath. "That's the whole of the school holidays."

"I know Kirk, but think about Zak. He's really excited. And it's the only chance he has of a proper holiday this year. I couldn't afford it on my own and you're not exactly much help are you?"

I grunted, knowing she was right but felt I had to make some sort of stand. "I was hoping to spend some time with him over Easter."

"Doing what Kirk? Bloody midget hunting?" The ex wife shook her head as she spat out the words.

"You've heard about that have you?"

"Kirk, you never cease to amaze me. What the hell has gotten into you for Christ's sake? You do realise you are going to end up being sectioned again don't you?" Her voice was as bitter as it was challenging. "Don't you ever think about how your son feels when he hears all this crap about his father?" She opened the window and reached for a cigarette.

"He knows then?" I asked quietly.

"*He* told me Kirk," she snapped, fumbling with a lighter that she couldn't get to work.

"I was half hoping he might tag along. He might enjoy himself."

The ex wife threw the lighter at the bin, shouting in exasperation at me and it. The sausage kings scarpered to the cover of their beds knowing the chance of food was highly unlikely. "Listen to yourself will you? Midget hunting. Do you honestly believe your son wants to be part of all your pathetic nonsense? He's twelve years old Kirk. He needs a father not some nutter who everyone takes the piss out of constantly."

"What is that supposed to mean?" I said, my interest piqued at this last statement.

"I hear it every day. So does Zak. His mates constantly poke fun at him about you. They look on your stupid CROUCHING thing on the internet all the time. Then I get questioned by the parents and on it goes. Oh believe me, everyone knows about you and your nonsense."

I sat silently, waiting for her to get it all off her chest. It was great news that the kids were taking so much interest in the CROUCHING community. Future blood.

"This midget hunt thing takes the biscuit," the ex wife carried on. "Do your parents know any of this?"

"Sorry?" I said when I realised she was expecting an answer. I had been mulling over the potential prospect of a 'Young CROUCHERS' group or something.

"Your parents Kirk. Do they know about this midget hunt thing?"

"I expect they soon will do. I have the Home Prevention Team coming around theirs today. That's why you have to drop me over there. Sinister sounding lot don't you reckon? The Gestapo of the mental health world."

"What?" The ex wife said shortly but obviously wasn't interested in listening to my explanation. She went on, "you really need to sort yourself out Kirk. You're getting worse if that's possible. Perhaps it's best that we *are* going away."

"What about the dogs?" I asked already knowing the answer.

"They're going in the kennels. It's just as well, knowing what sort of mood you're in."

She was right of course, but I didn't particularly want to see it that way. "It's like sending them to prison. They're my dogs too remember."

The ex wife was having none of it. "I've made my mind up. I'm dropping them up there tomorrow."

"Great," I muttered but didn't bother arguing. "Where is Zak anyway?"

"He's gone into town with mum to pick up some bits for the trip. I've told him he can spend some time with you tomorrow, although I'm beginning to regret that now."

"I'll be fine. Listen, just because I'm organising a midget hunt doesn't mean I can't take care of my son."

"Hark at yourself Kirk," the ex wife said shaking her head as she did so. "Midget hunt. It's ridiculous. You're 41 years old."

I nodded, "I know, I should have done it years ago."

"See what I mean? There's no chance of me ever having a sensible conversation with you."

"Alright," I said raising both my hands up in a conciliatory manner. "What time can I have Zak tomorrow?"

"You can come over about elevenish. What do you intend doing?" She crossed her arms with an expression on her face that dared me to come up with something outlandish. Outlandish to her anyway.

"I don't know to be honest. I'll think of something." It was a bit of a worry considering I hadn't been anywhere outside a couple miles radius in nearly three years.

"Just make sure it's nothing ridiculous Kirk. Try and have a nice day with him for once." She finally had managed to light her cigarette and added, "right, when I finish this I'll drop you over your mother's."

We barely said two words to each other on the short drive across Plympton but when we pulled up outside my parent's house the ex wife switched off the engine and turned to face me and her tone had softened. "Kirk, I know we're divorced and everything but I still care about what happens to you, you know. You've got to stop all these crazy ideas of yours and sort yourself out. I thought the medication was helping?"

"I'm fine," I replied honestly. "I just like different things than you."

"You like different things than everyone."

"Hardly," I smiled at her. "The CROUCHING community is the fastest growing knee bending concern in southern England." I noticed I changed the scale of my boast each time I made the comment. Last week it was Western Europe, last night the world, today it was southern England. Whichever one it was the ex wife did not appear impressed.

"Here you go again. I give up. I honestly give up. Just think about your son Kirk. Think about what all this is doing to him. And think about what an embarrassment you have become."

She really knew how to make me feel good about myself, however right or wrong she may be. "Okay," I said clambering out of the car. "On that warm note I am off to see the brain police." I slammed the door and she revved the engine and sped off. "Fucking midget fancier," I said through gritted teeth as I watched the small hatchback disappear around a corner.

The Home Prevention Team consisted of a nervous young man of about 25 who had a limp, damp handshake and a middle aged woman who appeared to have some sort of alopecia. That wasn't a good sign for someone like me and I immediately found myself staring at the bald patch just above her left ear. My parents joined us, mother insisting on making us all a cup of tea first, which I for one was desperate for as my hangover was still far from gone. The woman asked me a number of questions, all of which had become second nature to me over recent years. Had I taken my medication? Was I sleeping okay? Was I eating okay? Had I had any thoughts of self harm? Had I had any thoughts of harming others? Had I been hearing voices? (Yes, the ex wife's was still ringing in my ears) And so on. I looked across at my mother who was transfixed by all this as normal. She looked like she was watching some shocking thriller on the big screen. The one good thing about the episode with the ex wife was that it had, along with the hangover, subdued me somewhat and my answers were all reasonable and without any of the outlandish remarks I had made to Diane the day before. The only slightly uncomfortable part came when the young chap asked me about digging midget pits at Harewood House which caused my father to spit a mouthful of tea over himself.

All in all the twenty minute question and answer session was pretty painless and they appeared satisfied that I wasn't about to jump off a tall building or kidnap a traffic warden. They did however, inform me that they would be around to check on me at the same time the following day which was a pain considering the Zak situation but unfortunately they made it pretty much non negotiable. In the end they said they'd come a half hour earlier.

After they left I had a spot of lunch and was subject to a much more intense round of questioning from my mother who for some reason seemed to want to focus on the midget aspect. About ninety percent of her questions were completely irrelevant and often ridiculous but I tried to keep my calm and reassure her that I was fine. In the end it was my father who, as always, came to my rescue and put a stop to mother's relentless barrage. "Leave it to the professionals. They know what they're doing." He said to her not for the first time. I was touched though, by her constant worrying of her errant son and tried as always to reassure her as best I could.

"Mum, honestly, I'm fine. I was just having a laugh at the expense of Diane yesterday and it got out of hand."

"Well, he ought to be careful what he says," Telling my father rather than me which was often the way. "He'll end up in the funny farm again. Fancy saying you are going to dig holes in the ground for midgets to fall in." As usual she only got half of it right.

"Not for midgets to fall into mum, for us to throw them into when we catch them." The minute I said it I knew I would regret it and one look across at my dad who was shaking his head told me all I needed to know.

Mother sprang upright on her armchair. "What are you saying? Hunt them? No wonder these house protection people are after you."

"Home Prevention Team," the old man corrected but mother was like a dog with a bone now.

"I told you he shouldn't have moved in with that Emma." I didn't even bother correcting her. "She's just as bad and you know you can't drink on those pills." Tell me about it I thought. After a few more minutes of Gemma, Nikki, Craney, the ex wife et al being blamed for the midget problem I finally decided it was time to make my departure when the thyroid gland was brought into the equation. After a large reassuring hug and a promise to behave myself (whatever that meant) I left my mother looking happily concerned and got a pat on the back from my dad telling me that I knew where they were if I needed them. I walked quickly away wondering if he was in some way offering his services to the upcoming hunt.

The conversation with the ex wife was of *more* concern to me as I walked in the early Spring sunshine and I found myself weighing up the pros and cons of Zak disappearing to Italy for the Easter break. On one hand I was going to miss him, especially our nights in front of the box watching the football but on the other hand it would leave me in peace to concentrate of the midget hunt without him and the ex wife in the mix. I would miss the sausage kings but again, it would be useful not having to worry about them for a couple of weeks. Funnily enough my thoughts had moved on to Lucy; she was working for the first week of the kids school break but had the second off, when she rang me.

"Hello yes?"

"Hey you. My head hurts."

"Hello fat headed one. I was just thinking about you."

"Really? Where are you?"

"Just walking to the pub. I've survived my first session with the sinisterly named, Home Prevention Team." I heard Lucy laugh.

"That sounds painful."

"It was."

"How long are you staying at the pub?"

"Lord knows. Most of the afternoon no doubt. Football to watch, midget hunts to organise."

"Okay. I'll try and pop in. I've a few bits to do with the kids first. I presume when you say pub it's the Josh?"

"Just for a change," I confirmed, and then added, "I don't have any ham though."

There was a tutting sound in my ear. "That's just not good enough Kirk. I'm a high maintenance sort of chick."

"I suppose you're the type who expects Waitrose finest on the second fucking date?"

"At the very least. Right I have to go. I'll text you when I'm all done."

"Okay fat head" I replied and the call ended. The brief conversation cheered me up no end. I hadn't ever thought I'd be seeing Lucy again so soon. I walked the rest of the way to the pub with a smile on my face, my hangover finally lifting.

When I arrived at the pub I was pleased to see Craney and the rest of the lads who would make up the mainstay of the hunt were all stood at the bar, noisily conversing. Craney himself looked like he hadn't been to bed and for some reason big Andy was wearing a straw hat. I didn't bother to ask.

"About fucking time," boomed Carter. "We were about to send out a midget patrol to look for you."

"Yeah, I was worried you been picked up by the short arm of the law," added Lenny.

"Sorry chaps," I said truthfully. "In a manner of speaking my tardiness is midget related. The brain police wanted to grill me about my midget related opinions."

"Midget fanciers!" Shouted Carter and passed me a bottle of Pils. I took a gulp and waited patiently for the chorus of 'midget fanciers' to run its course as the rest of the bunch took up Carter's shout. Eventually I was able to say "right lads; let's get this midget hunting meeting started."

We moved to the large corner sofa, ten of us in all and went about discussing all the practicalities the upcoming hunt would entail. After an hour of much laughter and argument on the finer details of how to corner a large headed dwarf. (I was surprised how many ways there was) The meeting ended when Lenny spat a mouthful of beer over George the window cleaner; the result of Craney insisting he once fucked a black midget at an acid house party when he was high on Ecstasy. "She fucking loved it Lenny! I banged her whilst I danced. There was so much smoke in the place from those machine things that you couldn't see fuck all. Anyway, she was black as the ace of spades and less than three feet tall. It was easy. Best bunk up I've ever had in a night club."

It was big Andy that had given me a nudge about going up the road to Peacock's for our special Saturday afternoon CROUCH. I nodded my agreement and called the meeting to an end. In all, fifteen of us left the pub and made our way up The Ridgeway. Another half dozen joined us as we passed the Post Office Inn, smiles on their faces as they greeted us. As we got closer to the clothes shop I could see around twenty people milling about outside, students by the look of them, brightly dressed and excitable, phones and cameras at the ready to film our efforts. I walked straight to them and nodded a quick greeting to the three who had been outside Hall, Graves and Lee. In front of the sliding doors I turned and faced my expectant community.

"Welcome to today's special afternoon CROUCH outside Peacocks on The Ridgeway, Plympton. As this is something of a protest CROUCH you are all more than welcome to make various animal noises should you choose to do so." With that I went straight into a nice and easy straight forward 120 degree double knee bend CROUCH. As one, the community followed suit.

The pavement outside the shop was completely packed and no one was able to enter or leave it or indeed the shops on either side. It took less than thirty seconds for Craney to let out a loud moo and Carter to start barking like a dog with rabies. The students needed no encouragement to join in and within seconds of Craney's initial moo the street sounded like a cross between a farm and a zoo. Saturday afternoon shoppers stopped and stared at us, as did a couple of passing cars which lead to a long back up the one way street. I smiled as horns started to blare adding to the general disturbance. A minute or so later young Mr Jones appeared in the doorway, took one quick look in my direction then quickly vanished from view. I wondered if he had gone off to call the police. I certainly hoped so.

After another five minutes or so the noise levels had reached ever increasing levels. I looked around and saw at least forty people of varying ages and social backgrounds all CROUCHING as one and belching out a whole myriad of animal noises, from the regular – barks, moos, quacks, to the more obscure – I later found out that two of the students were doing beaver and aardvark impressions respectively whilst Gregg from the Post Office was attempting a fairly bad version of a polar bear's mating call, not that I knew what a good attempt would have sounded like. Whatever the various noises, the effect of them all combined to bring a true cacophony to the Saturday afternoon. I was proud of my community and knew that once more we had moved up another gear. Things were definitely heading in the right direction. When a bloke I only vaguely recognised pulled his BMW up onto the kerb and got out to join in with the CROUCH, making loud monkey noises at the same time, a shiver ran down through me. People were at last beginning to take CROUCHING seriously.

I waited a few more minutes before standing upright and raising my right arm into the air. I had to shout to make myself heard. "Thank you all for attending today's CROUCH outside Peacocks on The Ridgeway, Plympton. Tomorrow's Sunday morning CROUCH will take place outside the Woodford Methodist Church at ten past ten. I would also like to take this opportunity to remind you of next week's Good Friday midget hunt. All hunters are to meet outside the Sir Joshua Reynolds at 11 a.m. fancy dress optional but advised. Finally, don't forget to measure your children's heads on a regular basis." The last remark led to an outburst from Craney and Carter of 'water melon heads'

I was bombarded with requests from the students to have my photo taken with various threesomes and foursomes. Craney appeared by magic beside me, keen to have an excuse to mingle with a few of the pretty young things. He squeezed in between me and a striking looking spiky blond haired girl; taller than him and who had already caught my eye due to her bright pink Doc Marten boots and *very short* shorts. Craney suddenly remembered he had taken out his false teeth; for some reason he believed he could moo better without them and dropped them onto the ground as he fumbled in front of the tall blond punky student. She bent down and picked the plate up and handed it back to him. He made a hash of putting it back in his mouth and decided discretion to be the better part of valour and shot off back down the street. I made a shrugging gesture to the girl and she laughed, her teeth if possible were even whiter than Lucy's. Again, just as before, the thought of Lucy appeared to magically make my mobile ring.

"Hello yes?"

"Hey you."

"Ah fat head; you've just missed a truly wonderful CROUCH. One of the best yet."

"How very sad." Her voice had a thick slice of sarcasm in it.

"I'll tan your arse woman if you continue to be so insolent."

"Oh yes please." She mocked me. "I'm about ten minutes away from the pub."

"Okay. I'll walk back down there now."

"Peacocks?"

"Where else?"

"You are so predictable. See you in ten."

I said a few farewells to the remaining community, now mostly just the students, thanked them again for coming and along with Lenny wandered back to the pub. When Lucy arrived the bar was buzzing with excitement following the success of the CROUCH. I was basking in the glory of the biggest CROUCH yet. *And* it had only taken one day's notice. I could tell that things were beginning to really happen. My hard work was finally paying off. All those solo CROUCHES outside Hall, Graves and Lee on freezing cold Monday mornings were finally achieving payback. I was huddling at the bar with Carter and Lenny as Lucy tapped me on the shoulder. Turning, I had expected it to be Craney who I had just heard laughing but, no, there she was. And just like the night before, the sight of her took my breath away.

"Hey you," Lucy announced herself with a beaming smile lighting up her face.

"Hello fat head," I returned, stooping as I turned, to kiss her on the cheek. She smelt wonderful again. "You ought to have been here half an hour ago, you could have taken part in what will become known as the 'Peacock Farm' CROUCH."

"Is that all you lot ever go on about? Right my shout. Another Pils I assume?"

I nodded as she pulled a note from her small purse, which looked incongruous coming out of her huge hand bag. She saw me looking at it and laughed "A girl can never have a big enough bag."

I just nodded and stared at her arse as she turned to the bar. Her tight jeans definitely did her justice.

"Do you want a glass Kirk?" Lucy asked.

"What?" I had been caught out with my staring.

"A glass?" She pretended to ignore my ogling.

"Oh. Yeah. Sorry, I was staring at your arse."

"Twat."

"It's actually not bad for an old bird," I said seriously as she handed me my drink.

"Oi! Watch it mister. Oh yeah, while I think of it, that message you sent me last night was disgraceful." She tried not to laugh as she said this but failed miserably.

"You reckon?" I raised my eyebrows at her. I was always able to maintain a serious expression even in the most comical of situations.

"I know so."

We made our way to the same corner table I had sat earlier and I spent ten minutes telling in detail about what she had just missed outside Peacocks.

"You lot are really crazy. I can't believe forty people turned up."

"I know," I said nodding slowly, "I was expecting at least double that.

Lucy laughed and gently kicked me under the table and mouthed the word 'twat' before asking, "so you didn't get taken away by the men in white coats this morning then. How did it go?"

"Okay actually," I said smiling. "Although the old man nearly choked when they asked me about midget pits."

Lucy laughed loudly and shook her head. She was wearing her hair completely down today. It fell over her face and I found myself automatically reaching across and brush it from her eye. I kept my hand flat against her cheek and she reached up and touched it. Our eyes met and for a second I thought about saying something profound. In the end all I could manage was a rather pathetic, "you're skin is soft."

"Thanks," she answered as I took my hand away.

"I was expecting stubble."

"Twat," she broke out into that wonderful smile again. It had already implanted itself into my psyche and I found my heart speed up every time she did so. I told her about my earlier summons from the ex wife and Zak going off to Italy. She told me not to worry and said the break would do me good. I don't think she realised how much trouble I could get in to over a period of a fortnight. I kept that part to myself and again turned the subject of conversation around to her health issues. This time Lucy appeared a little more ready to open up. She knew I wasn't going to let her rest until she did.

"How long have you known?" I asked, seriously for once.

"About a year, off and on." Lucy looked down at her glass, appearing to not want to look at me.

"Why haven't you told me?" I was shocked to find out she'd known for so long.

"Because like everything else I just bury my head in the sand and hope it goes away." She made an expression that looked like she couldn't make her mind up about something. I didn't offer any help and just sat and waited for her to go on. After a few moments wetness came into her eyes so I reached forward and squeezed her hands. I still didn't say anything. Eventually she opened up. "I started getting pains in my chest, a bit like when you get a stitch. I didn't take any notice of it to be honest. I'm always getting aches and pains. Anyway, as soon as it came it would go again, sometimes for months. Then it came back really badly whilst I was at work. I went to the G.P. and had the usual tests, blood pressure, you know, that sort of thing and the nurse took some blood."

I couldn't help butting in at this point. "It wasn't yellow was it?"

"What?"

"Your blood. Was it yellow?"

"Shut up and listen," she said sternly, keen to get on with the story of her health now that she had started. "Anyway, the blood test came back with something or other and I had to have a load more taken. Then the doctor decided that I needed a bloody heart scan and I ended up in Derriford hospital having all sorts of stuff done."

"Fanny problems was it?"

"Will you shut up for five minutes Kirk," she snapped at me. "Of course the first thing my G.P. told me to do was cut out the fags and vodka until they found out what was wrong. And of course that just made me smoke and drink more."

"I don't suppose I help too much there do I?" I gave her a crazy grin.

"No you fucking well do not." She laughed, finally lightening up when she appeared to be on the verge of tears.

"So they told you, you had an irregular heartbeat?"

"Yeah, they found that out fairly quickly but what they can't figure out at the moment is why it comes and goes. If it was always irregular that would be fine. I say fine but, you know what I mean, they could work with that. But because it's not I continue to be tested on like a lab rat or something."

"You're not about to have a heart attack on me are you fat head?"

"That depends how excited you get me," Lucy replied winking at me mischievously.

"Fucking hell you'll be fine with me then," I laughed. "So what's happening next?"

Lucy shrugged, "God knows. I'm waiting to hear about the last lot of blood that was taken. I had a letter from the consultant saying I would hear before Easter but you know what they're like. It could be months."

"Have they given you anything in the meantime? For the pains?"

"No. They just said to stop smoking and cut down on the booze." She burst out laughing.

When she had stopped laughing I said in a serious manner, "I was going to offer you the wildest sex ever but obviously I will now have to withdraw the offer."

She kicked me under the table again, this time harder and said, "twat," just as I expected and then added that she 'needed a fag.' I raised my eyebrows to which I was told to 'fuck off' as she grabbed Carter who was also making his way outside for a smoke.

I got up and went to the bar to get another round in. Opening my wallet and pulling out my last twenty, I thought that it probably *was* best that Zak was pushing off for the Easter break. I really needed to curb my drinking costs a bit. By the time I was served and had got the drinks, Lucy had finished her cigarette and we sat back down at the same time.

"Your pals are all as crazy as you," she said shaking her head and pouring the leftover ice from her first drink into the one I had just placed down on the table.

"No one is as crazy as me fat head and don't you forget it. Nice fag?"

"Wonderful," Lucy replied then broke out into a cough.

When she had finished coughing I peered at her over the top of my glasses. "I like you fat head. I like you a lot. You've got a nice arse."

Lucy laughed and said back, "I like you to. You've got a nice..." She made an exaggerated point of looking me over. "...chin."

"Chin? You could have at least said smile or something."

"Okay, you have very nice green eyes. When I can see them that is."

"Of course you're right about my eyes. That's why I wear the dark glasses. If I don't I get swamped by women wanting me."

"You really are such a fucking twat," Lucy laughed

"I'm considering allowing you to come out with me again," I added, to which she aimed another kick at my shins. This one connected. "Shit. How pointy are your shoes?"

"Very," she said smiling. "And very high too." She slipped one off and held it up to show me. She was right about it. *Very* pointy and *very* high.

"Can I sniff it?" I made a grab for the black stiletto shoe but Lucy pulled it away from me at the last minute.

"My feet don't smell, thank you very much," she said somewhat primly.

"I won't bother then. Do you have any old trainers?"

"Will you fuck off?" Lucy screeched at me causing a few heads to turn in our direction. Then she thought for a few seconds and said, "of course I could always fill my boots with ham for you to feast on."

"Will you marry me fat head."

"FUCK OFF! And here I am thinking it was my *arse* you liked."

"Sorry fat head, you may have a pert behind but when it comes to ham there's simply no choice for me." I held my arms open to emphasise my decision.

"Do you know what? The worrying thing is that I think I believe you."

I smiled. "Ham is ham."

"You said it."

We carried on talking nonsense for a while, enjoying each other's company and happy to be able to not have to say anything too deep. To my huge surprise I found myself accepting Lucy's offer of a lift home when she announced that she better be leaving. I just didn't want to be apart from her and even the offer of a few minutes in her car appealed. What Lucy wasn't prepared for was me shouting "go left" or "next right" full blast each time we approached any junction. Eventually she pulled over to the kerb and shouted at me to calm down. "I don't go in cars very often," I said by way of explanation. "I get over excited." She called me a "twat" and pulled away slowly only for me to shout "reverse reverse" over and over until we got to Gemma's. A five minute journey ended up taking over twenty and when I asked Lucy if she wanted to come in and see Gemma for a quick glass of wine she needed no second invitation.

"Wow," Lucy exclaimed as she made her way down the steps to the front door. "Gemma told me you liked to bring her home gifts."

I stopped behind her and surveyed the pile of 'For Sale' signs and my latest offering – the gate. "It's a display of my affection," I said lightly, then added, "I know where you live."

Lucy turned to face me. "Don't even think about it."

"Well at least if a gate or something appears in your front garden, you'll know who put it there."

"I mean it Kirk." She gave me a suitably stern look.

I pushed past her and slid open the porch door and went inside. Gemma was just about visible behind a huge pile of ironing and with music blaring from the stereo system didn't notice either of us until I made her jump by peering over the pile of clothes and shouting 'boo!'

"Fucking idiot," she snapped at me but her expression instantly changed when she saw Lucy. She barged me out of the way and grabbed Lucy, giving her a big hug. They were like lost sisters who hadn't seen each other in years, not people who had only just met. Gemma was brilliant at making people feel welcome and she ushered Lucy into the kitchen and quickly poured her a large glass of red wine. Lucy tried to object to the generous measure but Gemma was having none of it. "Get it down you girl. And grab that packet of fags." She pointed to an open packet precariously balanced on the sink draining board. "Light one for me would you Lucy?"

The two girls smoked, drank and gossiped merrily away and I took the opportunity to check my voicemails; my phone had been buzzing away in my pocket for ages. I had two messages the first of which was from Craney, attempting to disguise his voice but failing miserably. He was trying to pass himself off as some kind of doctor, in an office that had a background noise of clinking glasses, rock music and Carter shouting something about 'nice tits,' I was informed that I had to have a full testicular cancer check due to their lack of use in the bedroom arena. The second message was from an Asian guy called Derek who wanted to speak to me about my credit card. That was considerate of him I thought.

By the time Lucy had plucked up the courage to tell Gemma that she really did have to leave I had hardly been able to get a word in edgeways. I felt genuinely sad that she was leaving and told her so.

"I like spending time with you too Kirk. You really do put a smile on my face." She reached up and kissed me on the lips. "Sorry if I don't taste of ham today," she smiled and gave me another quick kiss before turning to open to front door.

"One day I'll force feed you Marks and Sparks wafer thin and snog your face off," I said grabbing her before she could get out of the house.

"Can't wait. Now I really have to go Kirk."

I stopped her just as she was stepping outside. "At least promise me you'll come to the Sunday morning CROUCH?"

Lucy smiled and shook her head. "Sorry honeybun. Sunday mornings are swimming time with the girls. I've got my figure to think of, especially as I'm such an *old* bird." She blew me a kiss and went quickly up the steps to her car.

I watched the car pull away and then stared at the mess in the garden. Gemma appeared next to me, a topped up glass in her hand and followed my gaze. "What are you going to do with all of it?

"Admire it." I answered.

"Seriously Kirk? As much as I love your late night gifts they can't stay there forever. I've already had her next door moaning." She made a gesture towards the neighbour's house.

"Why don't you ever bring me home something useful?"

"Such as?"

"I don't know. Anything but fucking 'For Sale' signs."

"I got you a gate," I said looking at it lying haphazardly.

"And it's a lovely gate Kirk. But what the hell am I supposed to do with it?"

"I don't know. Paint it?"

"Fuck, you're mad."

I gave her arm a punch. "You wouldn't have me any other way."

"Damn right. Come on, it's getting cold."

We went back inside, Gemma to continue with her mountain of ironing and me to wind up the Chinese community. I sat down at the computer and watched a brilliant video of the earlier CROUCH which had been uploaded by one of the students. The highlight was when the camera panned around to Craney who could be seen to stop mooing and break out into a hysterical bark at an elderly couple as they walked past him. They both had a look of complete terror on their faces. I sent out a number of congratulatory messages and answered a dozen or more e mails. I ignored all the abusive messages from midgets and midget sympathisers, not wanting to give them any satisfaction of a reaction. Instead I made a post about the following day's CROUCH.

The Head of the CROUCHING Community would like to remind you all of tomorrows Sunday morning CROUCH outside the Woodford Methodist Church, Plympton at ten past ten. All denominations are welcome to attend but Chinese are excluded for obvious reasons. AND I will add that any Chinese trying to participate by using a disguise will be outted and have their feet measured accordingly. I would also like to use this opportunity to thank all of you who turned up for today's CROUCH outside Peacocks, which proved to be our most successful yet. Treat yourselves to some wafer thin ham, you deserve it.

Kirkland Christie   Head of the CROUCHING Community

I spent another half hour messaging my friends in New York who were threatening ever larger CROUCHES, looked at the photos of Lucy again and then spent the rest of the evening annoying Gemma and thinking about large headed dwarfs.

CHAPTER EIGHT

LIKE FATHER LIKE SON

CROUCHING Community Membership 3,649

The following morning after a good sleep I felt reasonably refreshed and was up and ready to go. I sent a text to the ex wife explaining that I had a session with the Home Prevention Team at eleven and would get the old man to drop me over to meet Zak straight after. I then had a quick bowl of cornflakes and three mugs of coffee one after the other, before marching off to the Woodford Methodist Church for my regular Sunday morning CROUCH. These always involved a venue with a religious element but because my agoraphobia limited the number of suitable locations many of these had been visited by me on a number of occasions; much to the dismay of the small congregations. I had even taken to CROUCHING outside old Vicarys, many of which were now private residences, much to the confusion of many a family having a Sunday morning fry up.

According to my watch I arrived dead on time and I passed through the open gate and

quietly slipped into a nice loose 150 degree double knee bend CROUCH. I never tried anything too complex on a Sunday. I held my position for about five minutes; nobody went in or out of the church and I didn't see one soul whatsoever pass by on the street beside me. In fact not even a car went by. This was more like the CROUCHING I was used to. I stood up and headed off to my parents in plenty of time for the brain police to ask their predictable questions. Nobody from all the various mental health people I had seen over the years had ever asked me the important questions, such as how much ham I was consuming or whether I considered sniffing full up dog shit bins a worthwhile pursuit. In one of my more 'reflective' moods I had spent three or four days visiting various dog walking areas and lifting up the lids on those red dog shit bins, having a long deep sniff. I waited for the sun to be on them to ensure maximum aroma. I had tried to get the lads involved but even they passed on this one. I must admit I had a little difficulty trying to explain its merits to Diane a few weeks later. Of course by they then the rain had come so it was hard for her to fully appreciate where I was coming from.

I arrived at my parents just in time for a coffee before the brain police arrived. This time the appointment only lasted ten minutes. I answered the usual questions and the balding woman confirmed my appointment with the psychiatrist the following day. The nervous looking lad who had come with her yesterday had been replaced by a nervous looking girl who managed to not say one single word during the whole meeting. So much for the men in white coats I thought. I silently praised Cameron's cut backs. The minute they were out of the door I got my father to shake a leg and managed to get to the ex wife's bang on eleven thirty.

Zak had decided he wanted to ride his bike to Plymbridge woods, a pretty valley a couple of miles to the north of Plympton where the river Plym coursed its way through from the heights of Dartmoor above. I knew the area intimately and considered it just about manageable on my limited radar. His plan was to hang a rope swing over the river and basically try not to kill himself. I still had an old mountain bike in the ex wife's garage which I had spent a small fortune on five years ago and ridden probably no more than three times. It was covered in dust but looked in reasonable condition. The ex wife passed me a ruck sack packed with food, explaining that it would only be thrown out before they left for Italy and twenty minutes after arriving there I was following Zak up the road admiring the huge piece of rope he had wrapped around the frame of his bike.

It was a fairly steep climb (by my standards anyway) to the crest of the hill, which was basically the skyline and border of Plympton, before the steeper descent down to Plymbridge itself. I was pleased to be able to freewheel down through the cool air but soon realised that the back brake blocks were about as close to the wheel as I was to a reunion with the ex wife. This left just the front brakes which were so sensitive even the slightest touch on the brake lever lead to me nearly going over the handle bar. Of course Zak found this hilarious and spent the whole downhill journey braking and skidding in front of me. It took me every threat of extreme violence to finally make him stop. In the end I had to use the soles of my trainers to help come to a stop and an incredibly muddy stretch of grass which left me absolutely thick with crap. After a few 'pleasantries' with Zak were exchanged and I had managed to just about prevent a cardiac arrest, we made our way along the popular cycle route until we came to the weir. The stretch of water behind it was deep enough to swim in and hadn't changed in the thirty years since I used to as a kid of Zak's age. In fact a group of us would often come here after school during the warm June and July afternoons. I tried to recall if Lucy had been amongst us but couldn't remember.

We were pretty much alone as we threw the bikes down on the grass, which like everything around us was a brilliant spring green. The trees overhanging the river were well on their way to reproducing this year's crop of new leaves and the only noise came from the huge number of birds going about their business of nest building and mate chasing. Zak appeared oblivious to all this and was busily edging around the bank of the river stopping every so often to dip a toe into it.

"The water's freezing dad," he said frowning.

"What do you expect son? It's come straight off the moors."

"It's ridiculous" The wonderful logic of youth.

I found a spot to sit and opened the rucksack to see what the ex wife had prepared for us. It was a veritable feast. Zak came over a grabbed a coke, managing to spray it all over me in the process of opening it and I poured myself a coffee from a large silver flask. We tucked into chicken legs and sausage rolls and decided on a plan of action.

"I can easily climb up that one dad," said Zak pointing across the river to a huge sycamore tree which had a couple of branches hanging enticingly over the river.

"There's no way you're going up there. You'll break your neck if you fall out."

"It's easy dad. I've climbed way bigger than that before." He wandered off to the edge of the river again to take a closer look. I shook my head and sat back, leaning against a small tree stump, enjoying the sun and the peace. I watched a couple of dragon flies zipping along the river, their bright shimmering bodies catching the streaks of sunlight that beamed through the gap in the trees like some strange alien light show. My mind turned to Lucy. It would be nice to have her here now, her head resting on my chest. I could even squeeze her head a bit if I was concerned at how short she was without her heels on. She would be swimming now, I guessed. I wondered how good she looked in her swimming costume. A lot better than me in my trunks I reckoned. Zak had started to throw stones into the river to see how deep it was. How he thought he would achieve this I had no idea but he seemed happy enough. Back when I was still with his mother we would almost always go off somewhere for the day on a Sunday and explore the coastlines of Devon and Cornwall. I used to find all sorts of beautiful hidden coves, well away from the tourist trails and Zak would spend hours being chased around by the sausage kings. It was nice to see that the sense of outdoor adventure was still instilled in him. If the dogs had been here now they would no doubt already be in the river swimming about with Zak trying to encourage them to get as close to the weir as possible. Nowadays this was about as far as it went for a day out for me. My once family filled adventures had turned into lonely CROUCHES outside boarded up shops and eight hour sessions of laying face down on the kitchen floor. How life had changed. A robin flew down to investigate my presence in his territory and I threw him a few raisins which he greedily swallowed one after the other. He flew off when Zak returned carrying the large rope.

"Dad, there's loads off fish in there," he said excitedly. "We should have brought my fishing rod."

"It's not like the sea mate; you need a license for rivers."

"That's crap Dad. I'm going in to get one." He removed his trainers and within seconds was wading out into the river staring downwards and shouting to me how cold it was. I watched him for a couple of minutes before getting up to consider the rope swing and where best to set it up. I walked over to Zak who had seen me holding the rope and had rushed to the edge of the river to point directions to me.

"That big one there dad," he called, pointing to a branch that already had the remnants of previous swings hanging limply from it. I could see it was the obvious choice.

"I'll climb up and you can throw me the rope," Zak said already making his way back across the water.

"Zak, you don't need to climb anything. We just throw the rope over the branch and tie a slip knot." I removed my trainers, socks and tracksuit bottoms and with just a bright green pair of shorts and T shirt slowly began to wade across to the other side of the river. Zak was right, it was absolutely freezing. The rain must have been falling heavily on the moors because it was a lot deeper than I expected. Just to add to the cold Zak had started to heave boulders at me causing the water to splash up all over me. The more I shouted at him the more he did it. Eventually I managed to pull myself up on the opposite bank and scramble over the thick scrub to the foot of the tree. After half a dozen attempts I managed a perfect throw and pulling the slip knot tight the rope swing was ready.

"You can go first dad. I'm not going to until you do." Zak was wading across towards me seemingly oblivious to the cold water which was up around his chest.

"Bloody chicken."

"You don't know how to tie knots."

"Well, we'll soon find out." I tied a couple of knots at the end of the rope to both shorten it and give me something to grip onto and gingerly scrambled up the steep slope for as far as I could. I smiled down at Zak below me who had now crossed the river and was edging along towards me, then ran down the slope and shouted "roundhouse!" for some reason as I leapt off the riverbank and swung out about twenty feet above the water. Just as I was thinking what a good job of the swing I had done, my hands slipped and I fell, back first into the water below, staring up at the branch above me as I did so. Fortunately the shock of the cold water only *nearly* killed me and helped compensate for the rush of air explode from my lungs as I hit the water twenty feet below.

"That was immense dad," I think Zak shouted to me as I tried to get the water out of my ears and waded back towards a desperately needed hot coffee.

"I'm glad you thought so," I tried to shout back, failing, but I think he got the general message. "And for Christ's sake stop throwing those stones!" Zak had begun another bombardment of me as soon as I had surfaced. Eventually I pulled myself out of the water and a few seconds later was stood shivering with a mug of sweet coffee cupped between my hands. I had finished it and poured another before Zak had gained the courage to finally take to the air. His previous six attempts had all been somehow aborted at the last moment. Unlike me however he ended up clinging hold of the rope like a man possessed and was left dangling high above the river.

"Dad, do something!" Zak shouted.

I threw a couple of stones at him.

"Dad you idiot! Help me!" I walked to the river bank and waited. He hung on for a surprisingly long time. Long enough for him to call me a whole host of things that were really quite unbecoming for a 12 year old. Eventually gravity won the standoff and he finally fell into the river. Unlike me once he was in the water he swam about happily and made his way back to the lowest part of the bank in order to go on the swing again. He emerged shivering but happy and shouted across to me, "that was brilliant dad, I'm having another go."

For the next half hour or so I watched Zak happily go in and out of the river, each time his confidence on the swing growing. Just as it looked like I was about to have to go for another plunge three lads a year or two older than Zak came along and immediately seemed interested in joining him on the swing. I was still absolutely freezing and was very relieved indeed to have a stay of execution. I had dug out Zak's towel and had used it to at least dry myself off a little but was already realising a change of shorts and T shirt would have been wise. I helped myself to more food and sat down in the sunshine and watched the four boys all having a great time. They quickly started to award each other marks out of ten for each crash into the water and soon they were even swinging two at a time on the rope. Although it was good to see Zak so obviously having fun, I felt a deep sadness run through me that there were so few days like this for me anymore. And in my heart I knew there wouldn't be that many to come. He was growing older and I was growing madder. He already found it difficult dealing with my condition and I was sure as he moved into his teenage years this would only become an even bigger issue. No amount of CROUCHING would replace my relationship with him.

I tried to rid myself of these thoughts, got up and wandered over to the river. "Boys, there's a load of grub and a drink over here when you're ready. It's all got to be eaten. They didn't need any more encouragement and a few minutes later I was handing out various sausage rolls, sandwiches and slices of quiche to shivering hands.

"How long can we stay dad?" Zak asked between mouthfuls of pork pie.

"I'm in no rush Zak. For as long as you can stand the cold."

I watched as Zak shared the food around with the other boys, pleased to see his generous nature was as good as it had always been. He even offered his towel to the older lads to use. The ex wife had always been very generous and fortunately most of Zak's characteristics were similar to hers not mine. Long may that continue, I thought. It would destroy me to see him end up like me. No wonder my father looked so sadly at me when he thought I didn't notice. He had witnessed his happy, successful and healthy son destroy himself and those around him in just a few short years. I tried to ignore these difficult thoughts entering my head and called out, "leave me at least a chicken leg lads." They were munching their way through the ex wife's feast like they hadn't eaten in a week. I poured myself another coffee and managed to grab a small pasty before it disappeared. Once the food had been demolished they trooped back across the river and continued to amuse themselves on the rope swing. I was always a great believer in getting your kids outdoors to play and surely this beat being sat on a Playstation in a dark bedroom all weekend. I had often used this reasoning to try and persuade the ex wife that CROUCHING was something Zak would benefit from but as always it fell on deaf ears. As I watched them begin the process of trying to manage all four on the rope at once it dawned on me that I was going to have to ride back in my wet shorts and T shirt or at the least in just my track suits bottoms. From past experience I knew I was going to end up with a raw arse. I saw that the ex wife had packed Zak a full change of clothes, right down to another pair of trainers should his get wet. Eventually the other boys left and Zak came over to me looking almost blue. I wrapped his towel around him and poured him the last of the coffee.

"It should be nice and warm in Italy," I said as he tried to stop his teeth chattering.

"Gran says it's over 70."

"Lovely. I wish I was going. You'll have a good time. Your Uncle Bob's mad. What I'll do is give you a ring over the Easter weekend."

"Yeah."

"Right, we best be packing up."

"Can we go on the bike path down to MacDonald's dad?"

I had been expecting Zak to say this. It wasn't a bad idea actually because it was flat all the way and I was already worrying about my potential arse problems. "Yeah, I don't see why not. Just give your mum a text when you get some reception and let her know where we are okay? " He nodded and wrapped the towel around him in order to change his clothes. "Are you seriously still hungry?"

Zak nodded, "I'm starving dad."

I shrugged and got everything together and gingerly sat on my bicycle. I knew I was going to pay for this tomorrow. The ride was a couple of miles at the most and didn't take long at all. For once I didn't have to worry about my brakes and Zak seemed happy to trundle along without trying to annoy me. However, by the time we got to MacDonald's my arse was already beginning to feel raw and I winced as I climbed off, handing Zak a fiver to get himself the cheeseburger and fries he was so desperate for. I hated the stuff and just told him to get me a coffee. Recently I seemed to be eating less and less which wasn't a bad thing but according to my shrink wasn't a particularly good thing either. It wasn't like I was starving myself or anything. I just didn't feel particularly hungry. Food was over rated anyway. I have always believed that a good diet would include a bout of prolonged mania. Fat women everywhere would shed stones in a couple of weeks no problem.

"Have you got a monkey arse dad," Zak said handing me my coffee and breaking me from my fat thoughts.

"I can feel a baboons ring coming on. I'll be walking around like I've shit myself tomorrow. Listen mate, I haven't got much cash to give you," I said handing him about £17.

"Don't worry dad, Grandad's giving me some money and I still have about £50 from my birthday left."

"Yeah but if I had known I could have put a bit back. You know I don't get a lot." This was true. My £50 a week disability allowance went to the ex wife and the other £70 was basically used to supply me with everything else, mostly booze. Gemma got my housing benefit paid straight into her account and I still bought her a few bottles of wine and a pizza or something each week to help out. I really needed to get a grip and get a job. Although who would employ me I had no idea? I did get a driving job about eighteen months ago which ended in me falling asleep at the wheel early one morning due to the effects of my medication and that was the end of my job and my driving license. Since then I would say I was pretty much unemployable. In any case I had my CROUCHING community to consider. This was a full time occupation by anyone's standards. Anyway, I wished it was me taking him on holiday but we both knew this wasn't going to happen for a long time yet. At least we'd shared a good afternoon together without any disasters, bar my arse and I was happy to have had some quality time with my son. I had even managed to not embarrass him for once

I was resigned to pushing my bike back to the ex wife's and was taking ever shorter steps with an ever wider gait. I must have looked like John Wayne. Zak rode his bike around me calling me 'monkey arse' before finally tiring of my snail like pace. He gave me a wave and shot off up the hill no doubt getting home about half an hour before me. By the time I did make it back to the ex wife's I was dreaming of laying face down on the kitchen floor with a load of slices of freezing cold ham covering my arse.

Zak was already in the shower when I walked in the front door after putting the bike back in the garage. The ex wife put the kettle on and seemed in a fairly conciliatory mood for once. I think out of relief that I had managed to spend a day with Zak that he actually enjoyed rather than come home moaning about how I had embarrassed him. I had finished my drink by the time he came back downstairs demanding to see my red behind. I managed to fend his demands off and gave him a big hug and wished the two of them an enjoyable holiday before heading off on my slow trek back to Gemma's. The martyr in me had refused a lift and I was able to feel painfully sad to my heart's content as I trudged along the quiet streets. It had been a good day but it just brought back the memories of how life used to be. I had a good excuse to stop for a couple of lengthy leans and the fifteen minute journey took closer to an hour.

As soon I got to Gemma's I went up to the bathroom to inspect the damage. I pulled down my tracksuit bottoms and peered around over my shoulder into the mirror. A baboons ring indeed. I searched the bathroom cabinet for some form of relief and found a tube of Savlon. I gingerly applied it, washed my hands and went downstairs to lay face down on the kitchen floor. The house was empty and quiet and I had thirty minutes of contemplative lino sniffing before I heard the front door open and the sound of the girls' feet running along the hallway towards me.

"Mum! Kirk's lying on the kitchen floor again!" They both squealed in unison, followed by, "are you feeling sad again Kirk?"

"I've got a sore bum," I said without moving, which made them both laugh.

Gemma appeared carrying an inordinate amount of shopping bags which she dropped down around me. "Get up you nutter," she said and stamped a foot on my arse.

"Ow! Mind my baboons ring," I moaned and got up onto my feet.

The girls shrieked stuff about monkey bums before finally relenting and disappearing upstairs. Gemma ignored my moans and groans, busily emptying the shopping bags, so I grabbed her and said, "look at it Gem." I went to pull down my trousers to show her the damage but she grabbed my hands to stop me. "I'll take your word for it Kirk."

Ten minutes later I showed her anyway.

CHAPTER NINE

I ASKED FOR A 69 NOT A 99

CROUCHING community membership 3,997

"*Fuck me* mate, it's really taking off."

I had summoned Gemma to the computer to look at a video of the Times Square CROUCH in New York. There were easily over 100 people taking part; almost solely youngsters whom I presumed were Molly's student crowd. The community had arrived in the very centre of Manhattan just as Molly had promised. She had certainly done us proud.

"The CROUCHING gospel is spreading across the world. Soon we will be unstoppable."

I watched the clip over and over, scanning for any yellow faces amongst the throng. Molly wasn't nearly as anti – Chinese as me for some reason and I knew for a fact there was a large Chinese population in New York. I had argued with her before when she had broken my strict rules and she said that she couldn't persecute any of her friends. Also there was the added problem that there was quite a number Korean and Vietnamese CROUCHERS involved and from my view point they all looked the same. Without the advantage of seeing their fanny's it was impossible for me to make an informed choice. However, on this occasion there appeared to be no obvious Chinese look-alikes so I finished my inspection and messaged Molly my congratulations. The CROUCH in New

York showed how quickly numbers could grow given the right environment and commitment and it also acted as a nudge to me that I needed to pull my finger out over here. Molly was a 'big deal' in the student world and could easily raise plenty of numbers; her buddies no doubt thinking the whole thing a bit of a lark and just the sort of thing as students; they should be taking part in. I wondered whether any of them, including Molly herself, would ever feel the passion I did. Probably not. Actually never. Of course they wouldn't. To me CROUCHING was a way of life. Still, I liked the idea of tapping into the student population. The last few CROUCHES, especially the one outside Peacocks had seen a sharp increase in student attendance. God knows how they suddenly became aware of the community but the internet is a wonderful thing and I could see a real opportunity opening up to grow numbers quickly.

I was distracted by a message from a member in Liverpool that pinged up on the screen. It said that he had gone to his local Spar shop and in a similar situation to what had happened in Plymouth city centre; he had found that there was no wafer thin ham on the shelves. I could understand his outrage and messaged him back straight away encouraging him to organise a boycott of the shop and sent a link showing footage of my own recent protest. The idea of shop boycotting really appealed to me; I could see a lot of potential in it and made a mental note to look at various shops to picket outside once the midget hunt was over. I then made the following post on the community home page:

The head of the CROUCHING community would like to commend all of our New York members for such a wonderful CROUCH in Times Square today. CROUCHING activity continues to grow at a rapid rate across the world (except China) and it is this sort of commitment from Molly and her friends that show what can be achieved. Saying this, due to arse related injuries and further demands from the psychiatric world; my regular Monday morning CROUCH outside the spiritual home of CROUCHING Hall, Graves and Lee has had to be cancelled. Instead I shall be having my head examined followed by a couple of hours lying face down on the kitchen floor with numerous pieces of cold wafer thin ham on my bottom.

We are now less than a week away from the Good Friday Midget Hunt, so keep your eyes open; your children's head's measured and ALWAYS check under your bed before you turn off the lights.

Kirkland Christie   Head of the CROUCHING Community

I was considering turning in for the night when Lucy came on line.

'Hey you'

'Hey fat head'

'Sore arse? Dare I ask?'

'Not all of us are filthy like you. Actually it's a riding problem...saddle rash'

'LOL. I can't imagine you on a bike'

'Don't worry; I won't be again in a hurry. I can barely walk'

'Thought you were putting some ham on it'

'Ah, glad to see you are finally understanding the benefits of ham'

'I actually bought a couple of packs of wafer thin ham today'

'Good girl. You know what? I'm beginning to think you're alright after all'

'Twat'

'I've got the big shrink tomorrow'

'I know, what time do you finish'

'Not sure...late morning probably'

'OK ring me when you get out and we can do lunch if your arse is up to it'

'Sounds good'

'Right gotta go old man on a mission'

'Anal?'

'FUCK OFF!!!!!!!!!!!!'

'Laters xx'

'xxxx'

The following morning I was up and at them early. I ate a bit of breakfast; toast and ham, and waved Gemma and the girls off to her sister's. Some sort of zoo visit apparently. I cleared up, left the house and walked under overcast skies to my appointment with the psychiatrist. Normally I would be totally pissed off at missing my Monday morning CROUCH at the spiritual home of CROUCHING, especially for an appointment with the shrink, but the thought of lunch with Lucy cheered me no end. I stopped a couple of times for some off the cuff kerb jumping but couldn't quite get into it. Even with lunch with Lucy looming I was still a bit down with Zak going away and with my sore arse which was still throbbing with every step.

I found myself dwelling on the Zak situation as I made my way to the hospital. It was an area of my life that deeply troubled me and one that I just couldn't seem to get to grips with. It filled me with sadness when I thought of all the things in his life I had missed in the last few years. My sadness wasn't your normal sadness either. It was a deep hollow emptiness that I carried around with me like a dark cloud hovering over my head. No matter what I did or how much I tried I knew that the dark cloud was never too far away. Sometimes I would see it on the horizon, distant but there, ominous, waiting. At other times it would be right overhead, drenching me with its misery. The rain of dread and despair. Wherever the cloud was and wherever I was, the two of us were never far apart. If I won a million pounds on the lottery tomorrow the cloud would still be there, maybe hiding behind a building or a hill, but always there. My shrink had once told me that the things that bring the most happiness often brought the most misery. Probably more psychiatric bullshit. Take CROUCHING for example, I loved that and it had never brought me anything but pleasure.

The old man was waiting for me in the hospital reception. He had insisted on coming in with me which was both nice on his part but slightly disconcerting on mine.

"How are you feeling?" He asked patting me on the back.

"I'm alright dad. A bit pissed off that Zak's gone away at such short but okay other than that."

"There's nothing you can do about that," replied my father. "He'll have a good time and it gives you a chance to sort your head out while he's away."

I grunted. "I know, but it winds me up that nobody ever tells me anything until the very last minute just in case it sends me crazy." I put a finger to my temple as I said 'crazy.'

"It's a cross you have to bear I'm afraid."

We didn't have long to wait and I was soon sat in front of an old chap who looked exactly how I would have said a psychiatrist should look; a frizzy mop of white hair, huge bushy eyebrows and a pair of half rimmed old fashioned spectacles which he was peering over expectantly. He explained he was a locum as my usual shrink was away elsewhere and he asked the standard opening question that all shrinks seemed to ask: "so what is it that you think is wrong with you?"

Now there was probably a dozen or more replies I could have offered, in fact I nearly said that I was worried about a new plague of 'club foot syndrome' but I managed to refrain from it and answered, "I don't know. My psychologist made the appointment."

The elderly doctor smiled and tapped a few keys on the computer in front of him. He looked about as comfortable using a computer as I did eating chop suey. After a number of oaths under his breath and one final thump of the keys he gave up and turned back to me and said calmly, "I've never liked these things. Right Mr Christie at least I have your file to hand." He flipped open a brown folder and peered at some pieces of paper for a few seconds. "Right, I see you're on quite a cocktail."

I liked this doctor. He didn't appear to have any idea about the midget pits etc. What a stroke of luck I thought and said, "Yeah, but the combination seems to be working." Then I answered the usual eating, sleeping etc questions for the third time in as many days. If the old man wasn't with me I reckon I could have been in and out in five minutes but he went and chipped in about the concerns of my elevated mood. The shrink tried the computer again but gave up and instead asked me what had happened.

"Well I always have a bit of fun with Diane, my psychologist. She loves to take everything I say seriously. That's why I do it. Christ, if everything I told her was true I would have been in a straight jacket by now."

"What sort of things?" The shrink asked calmly.

"Oh, the usual for me. Stuff about the Chinese, it's become a standing joke. And I was laughing about midgets. I saw one the night before. I can't help it if I find them funny. Loads of people do." Fortunately my father did not embellish my explanation. The doctor didn't ask any other questions but just spent a few minutes flicking through the file. Eventually he put it down and said matter of factly, "right Mr Christie, here's what we're going to do." He scribbled some notes and then handed me a prescription slip. "I think we ought to reduce your Venlafaxine down to 150mg from your current 225mg. Just to be on the safe side. You're on a pretty big dose of anti depressants and if we aren't careful this could push your mood up too much. I think dropping them back a little should ease the chances of this." Great, I thought. It's like they don't want me to be happy. The shrink went on, "I'm going to leave everything else the same until you see your normal doctor next month. I'll make sure someone rings you with an appointment date." He passed me the prescription slip. "Collect these today and start taking them straight away. The best thing is to take all the 225mg pills back to the chemist." Five minutes later I was back outside with my father and thinking about another visit to the fat chemist.

"That was short and sweet," the old man said as we walked slowly over to his car.

"You never get long with the psychiatrist," I replied looking up at the sky to see if rain was likely. "I think I'll walk up to the chemist dad, seeing as the weather's okay." We said our goodbyes with me promising to keep in touch and to 'behave' and I headed off to see the fat chemist. I sent Lucy a text which just said 'ring me now' and was walking through St Mary's churchyard when my mobile buzzed in my jeans pocket.

"Hello yes?"

"You summoned me oh master."

"I'm all done."

"Where are you?"

"In St Mary's graveyard. Near the 'Fanny' grave."

"What?"

"There's a gravestone of someone called Fanny. Everyone knows that. We used to shout 'Fanny Fanny Fanny' at it on the way to school every day." This was indeed true.

"What school?"

"Old Priory juniors."

"You really are a twat Kirk. If I were you I'd go in the church and say some prayers. Your soul definitely needs saving."

"Funny fucker."

"Oi."

"Right, enough of churches and fannies. You don't hear that said together very often do you?" I heard Lucy laughing in my ear. "What time are we hooking up?"

"Well I've managed to get a long lunch so shall we say about a quarter to twelve?"

I looked at my watch. It said ten past ten. I looked over my shoulder at the church clock. That said twenty past four. "Fucking clocks," I said under my breath then to Lucy asked, "where do you want to meet?"

"How about the George?"

"No problem, I'll be there in plenty of time," I answered, having no real idea of what the time actually was. The George was a perfect choice. I may even see crazy Terry in there again. Lucy would love him.

I decided to give the fat chemist a miss for the moment, I didn't want to be late for Lucy and I headed off up the hill towards the George. I stopped at Peacocks and peered in through the window but there was no sign of Mr Jones. I gave it a couple of minutes but gave up, keen as I was to see Lucy. However, I was delayed when Carter came out of Barclays bank and shouted a subtle "Christie you Nonce!" across the road at me. I walked over to him and he didn't look happy.

"Alright mate? I asked. "You don't appear in the best of moods."

"Fucking banks," he barked at me, his expression one of thunder.

"Do you want me to organise a CROUCH outside it?"

"Definitely. A fucking loud one." He didn't go into why he was so pissed off and I didn't enquire.

"All ready for Friday?"

He nodded and broke into a smile; the thought of the midget hunt instantly cheering him. "Oh yes indeed. I got the trombone out of the loft last night and gave it a good polish."

"I never knew you played one." I said instantly liking the idea of Carter blasting away on it.

"I don't. Haven't a fucking clue actually. It's my sister's old one. Fuck knows how it ended up in my loft but it's going to have an outing on Friday."

"Brilliant mate. I have Gemma's kid's bugle still. The one I had on New Year's Eve." The last New Year's Eve had been one of the more 'original' ones of recent years and had seemed to go on for days.

"We'll blast out the little buggers. Craney has at least three air horns apparently."

We laughed and chatted for a few minutes before I told him I was off to meet Lucy for lunch.

"The old ham ploy did the trick then mate?"

I nodded. "Never fails. Every bird's a sucker for a bit of the old wafer thin."

"Except the Jewish ones," laughed Carter. "And you don't want to be taking one of them to lunch do you? She'll even make you pay for her parking."

I left the subtle as ever Carter to his happy brand of humour and carried on up the hill to meet up with Lucy. The pub was surprisingly busy for this time of day and there were already a couple of groups of people milling around in the bar, ordering drinks before going through to the restaurant. I ordered myself a bottle of Pils for a change and took it outside to the benches which looked down at the main road below. I had been sat less than two minutes when Lucy went past in her car, not noticing me and turned into the car park around the back of the pub. I walked around to meet her and she pulled up in front of me smiling. I opened the door for her and my eyes went from her wide smile swiftly down to her legs which were on clear display. I had forgotten she would be dressed in her work gear. Helping her out she laughed when she caught me admiring her shapely pins, graced as always by a pair of shockingly high heeled shoes.

"Hey you," she said in her usual happy greeting and grabbed hold of me to kiss me on the lips. As usual she smelt wonderful.

"Nice legs fat head," I quipped, breaking free of her embrace and looking down at her legs once more.

"I don't live in jeans," she laughed. "If I knew I'd get such approval I would have worn one of my shorter skirts." The one she was wearing was already pretty short.

"From now on you are banned from wearing jeans in my company ever again."

She raised her eyebrows, lighting a cigarette at the same time. "I suppose the knickers and bra have to go too?"

"Don't be disgusting woman. What do you take me for?"

"A strange sort a pervert."

I shrugged. "Probably; in a ham related sort of way. You do realise I have a lino fetish don't you?"

She took a long drag on her cigarette and sat down at the table. "I *know* I'm gasping for a fucking drink."

"The usual?" She nodded.

I went inside and asked a young, pretty waitress about a table. She told me that all of them were reserved but we could sit in the bar. When I passed on this news to Lucy she didn't appear particularly perturbed. "Is Gemma home?" she asked taking a sip from her glass then reaching for her cigarettes again.

"Why? Are you going to cook for us?"

"Is she home?" She asked for a second time.

"No, she's gone to a zoo or something with her sister."

"Right, let's go to yours then." She put the unlit cigarette back in the packet and took a large gulp of her drink.

"We've got plenty in," I said. "Gem did a big shop yesterday.

Lucy removed my glasses and looked at me. "You really are such a twat Kirk. I'm not hungry. Not for food anyway. Comprendez?"

"Oh, right I see." I blurted out suddenly feeling queasy.

She ignored my somewhat reserved response and stood up, pulled me up also and led me to her car. When we were sat inside she leaned over and kissed me. Even without my glasses which Lucy still had hold of I couldn't help getting a good eyeful of her thighs as her skirt rode up extremely high, almost to her crotch. Unfortunately, as Lucy's tongue pushed itself into my mouth, *my* crotch didn't stir even a twitch. "Fucking pills," I tried to mutter as Lucy continued to 'snog my face off' as she would later call our first proper embrace.

"What?" She said a little breathlessly finally releasing me from her grip.

"Nothing fat head," I answered, wondering and worrying what the next couple of hours would bring.

"Do you have to keep calling me that?"

"What, fat head?" I said then added, "fat head".

"Yes, that. Can't you call me Lucy for once?"

"Sorry fat head. It's that or nothing at all."

Lucy started the car and I fastened my seat belt. "I think I'd prefer nothing at all then."

"Okay fat head. And anyway, at least mine's not a swear word like twat."

"Well you are a twat."

"And you fat head are a fat head."

We drove in silence for a while before pulling up at a red light for a pedestrian crossing, at which point Lucy turned to me and blurted out, "I think I'm having a breakdown."

"Me too, let's run off to Northampton."

Lucy burst out laughing. "Why Northampton?"

"I've no idea."

As the lights changed she reached over and squeezed my hand before changing gears. "Kirk, I'm being serious. My head's all over the place. I had a massive bust up with my sister in law this morning before I left for work. She rang me and started lecturing me about my stupid fucking husband. The kids are siding with him as always. Even my own mother has been having a go. You wouldn't believe I might have something seriously wrong with me." Her words came pouring out in a torrent and I held my breath as she just missed knocking a young lad off his push bike.

"With your heart and my brain we could make sweet music," I said a little lamely in an effort to lighten the mood.

"Are you ever serious about anything?" She said testily.

"Ham."

"For fuck's sake Kirk!" She shouted.

"Sorry fat head. I really don't know what you want me to say. You haven't said much at all about your heart problems and you didn't even mention it until the other day."

"I know and I'm sorry. I just didn't want you to worry about it. You've got enough problems with your own shit." She swore as someone pulled out in front of her even though she was driving way over the speed limit.

"Listen to me fat head; I thought you and me had a deal? I tell you about all my crazy shit and you moan to me about how crap your life is. You should have told me about your heart stuff. I am allowed to care about you." It was my turn to do the hand squeezing.

"I know. I'm sorry." She wiped a tear from her eye. "Shit, now I'm bloody crying. I don't do crying. What have you done to me?" She laughed and rubbed her eyes as we pulled up in front of Gemma's.

"I bring all my women to tears eventually."

"Twat."

We sat in silence for a few seconds before I said, "no more burying your head eh?"

Lucy smiled, her face slightly flushed. "You know I always will. I'm the ostrich of the family. I just slap on a bit of lippy, smile and say everything's fine."

"Have you considered class A drugs?"

"Yeah, many times and they didn't work either. Right come on I'm *hungry*." She made a big show of licking her lips.

"Are you sure you don't fancy going down to St Mary's and CROUCHING outside the west entrance?"

"You do make me smile Kirk. Now hurry up and take me to your lair," Lucy said making a naughty expression before adding, "I hope your sheets are clean."

"Not for long," I said slamming the car door and grabbed Lucy's hand, escorting her down the steps.

"Naughty boy," she said and winked at me as she pushed past through the open the front door.

I followed her through to the kitchen and grabbed a couple of bottles of Carlsberg from the fridge. As I searched for a bottle opener Lucy opened the fridge again, took a slice of ham from an open packet and rolled it up like a cigarette. She then slowly moved it in and out of her mouth replicating what I presumed to be a blow job.

"That's the sexiest thing I've ever seen," I said honestly.

"Twat," Lucy replied, swallowed the ham in one, blew me a kiss and said, "Come on, let's go to bed."

"What about the rest of the ham?"

"Fuck the ham. No change that, forget the ham, fuck me." She burst out laughing and pulled me to the staircase.

I followed her nervously up the stairs, at the same time finding myself thinking how sexy her legs looked in her short skirt and high heels. "I'm going to let it slip just this once but never ever abuse ham with such words again."

"Come on, before I change my mind." She pulled me into the girls' bedroom then burst out laughing. "I need the bathroom first anyway." I pointed toward the bathroom then went into Gemma's bedroom and told her not to be long. Once she'd closed the bathroom door I went down the landing to my own room, stripped down to my boxers, sprayed some aftershave over me and climbed under the duvet, cursing as I realised I'd managed to spray some of my Armani smelly on my 'japs eye.' I eventually stopped swearing and lay back on the pillows and stared up at the ceiling, very aware of how flaccid my manhood was. A few minutes later I heard Lucy shouting something about how I was a "total fucking twat." When she came in still telling me what a twat I was I didn't turn to look at her but continued to stare at the ceiling, my heart feeling as though it was about to burst through my chest. Suddenly I felt Lucy's warm body slide in beside me.

"Hello handsome boy," Lucy said softly rolling over onto her side to face me. I leant forward to meet her and kissed her, this time passionately enjoying the sensation of being lost in the moment. She closed her eyes and wrapped her arms around me, her leg hooking itself over my body. The kiss seemed to be going on forever. How long did these kisses last for? It had been such a long time since I had been in this position. What I did know was that despite being in the middle of a passionate embrace with an incredibly sexy naked woman, the stirring in my special area registered a big fat zero. I decided there and then that I would never take another pill ever again; not one from the fat chemist anyway.

I decided that the best thing I could do was use a diversion tactic, so I broke off from the kiss and rolled on top of Lucy. I began kissing her neck and whispering how beautiful she was in her ear. A nice touch I thought, even though I meant it. I slowly moved down to her breasts, which were really large in comparison to her tiny figure but were still wonderfully firm. I licked and kissed her nipples, which instantly hardened as my tongue caressed them. Lucy let out a small gasp as I sucked on one nipple and squeezed the other. Her sharp nails dug into my back and she whispered to me, "harder." For a moment I panicked before I realised she wasn't referring to my soft cock but in relation to my 'nipple attention'. I obliged and the gasps got louder. After a couple of minutes I turned my attention further south and for the first time noticed a bright red stone shining in a belly button piercing. I gently kissed it and moved slowly down to her black thong. Her hands were already pressing on the top of my head but I teased her for a few more minutes, kissing and licking around her underwear. At last I pulled the tiny thong to one side and buried my face in her most private of parts. The first thing I noticed was that she was either a lot younger than I thought or she'd had a good shave that morning. The next and more reassuring thing was that her fanny appeared to be going in the right direction. No hint of Chinese *sidewaysness* whatsoever. I went about my business like a man on a mission, determined to at least allow Lucy to get some pleasure before my predicament became obvious. Lucy's moans got louder and her fingers kneaded my hair and scratched my back in no particular order.

After a while my mind drifted inevitably to the midget hunt. After the all clear from the shrink and with the ex wife a thousand miles away, coupled with the obvious enthusiasm from the lads as shown by my earlier chat with Carter, it was shaping up to be a fantastic day. I wondered where the little bugger who had punched me in the nuts lived. I'd have loved to smoke her out, so to speak. Lucy let out a long stream of expletives which I took to mean she was reaching the point of no return. I winced as she really went to town with her nails on my back but put my tongue into overdrive as I felt her body stiffen and twitch and finally relax. She pulled me up to her and kissed me deeply, seemingly enjoying the taste of herself.

"Yummy," she exclaimed as if reading my thoughts.

"Dirty girl," I said, smiling down at her but already beginning to worry about what would happen next.

"Very," she said and kissed my again.

The inevitable eventually happened and I felt every part of my body stiffen except the bit that counted, as Lucy's hand reached down to my soft cock. There was no other way to describe it. Soft cock. It said it all.

"Oh dear," Lucy said and looked up at me with an expression that I couldn't work out. Was she sympathetic or mocking me?

"I'm sorry fat head; you just don't turn me on."

"Twat," she said smiling but unsure as to what to do next.

"Medication side affect I'm afraid," I said matter of factly. "That and your terribly smelly undercarriage have just ruined any chance of me getting my rocks off."

Lucy to her credit burst out laughing and wrapped her arms tightly around me and said, "hey, don't worry about it. I can wait."

"I decided when I had my head between your legs that I am stopping all forms of medication forthwith. In ten months time I will be fucking you like a battering ram."

"It's okay Kirk, you don't have to say anything. I'm not going anywhere."

"Except to the shower to wash that stinking monstrosity between your legs."

"Fuck off. You really know how to make a girl feel good don't you?"

This time I laughed. "You know I'm only pulling your leg fat head. Actually I think it was your arse I could smell not your fanny."

She dug her nails into my back as hard as she could, causing me to yelp. "Kirkland Christie, you really are the floppiest cocked twat I have ever met."

I rolled off of her and we lay beside each other, Lucy's leg wrapped tightly over me, one hand stroking my hair, the other stroking my soft cock. I thought about which church I should CROUCH outside on Easter Sunday. It really ought to be St Mary's. After a while she broke the silence and said, "you really have the strangest eyes. They're so green it's like they're not real."

"How do you mean?"

"I don't know. It's almost like you're looking right through me."

"Into your very soul." I said in what I hoped was a sinister voice, but probably sounder like the bloke from the X Factor. "And it's very very black,"

"That wouldn't surprise me."

"Lucy, I mean fat head; I am really quite fond of you."

"Ha! You called me Lucy. Then you fucking ruined it by saying your *fond* of me." She stressed the word fond.

"From me, fond is a huge compliment."

"Yeah right. I can't believe I'm laying here with you and not feeling one bit guilty whatsoever."

"You mean for forcing me to do that terrible thing to you?"

"Oh fuck off and kiss me you twat."

I did as I was told and when Lucy finally broke for air she said she had better be getting herself together. I nodded in agreement. "Yeah, you've taken up way too much of my time. I haven't even had my ham rations yet."

"You and fucking ham, you're obsessed."

"Probably," I answered admiring her wonderful body as she climbed from the bed.

She stopped before she went through the door and turned back to face me. Her tits looked fabulous and she waited for me to stop ogling them. "I need you in my life Kirk. I need to spend lots and lots of time with you."

"I need you too fat head. You've become very very special to me, even if you don't turn me on in bed."

She turned and stomped off to the bathroom shouting, "you're such a fucking twat" over her shoulder as she did so.

CHAPTER TEN

UNCLE PERCY AND HIS UNFEASIBLY LARGE SHOE

CROUCHING Community Membership: 4,402

I stayed in bed for an hour after Lucy left to return to work. I felt somewhat relieved to have survived the first hurdle of my sexual problems and knew that now the decision had been made to stop taking my medication it would not be long before I arrived at the second hurdle; good old Uncle Percy. I had been taken completely by surprise by Lucy's sudden decision to take me to bed, but now I knew our closeness and dependence for one another had been sealed, even if I had not been up to the task so to speak. A few minutes after hearing her car pull away I got a text from her telling me she now saw it as her duty to make me hard and for the first time in Lord knows how long, I was actually looking forward to letting someone try.

   Twelve hours later I was sat in front of the computer deep in conversation with my American friends about their recent CROUCHING exploits, safe in the knowledge that there was absolutely no chance of me getting any sleep that night due to my knew non – medicated state. I was on Skype listening to Molly as she told me about her latest plan for an even larger CROUCH on Fifth Avenue or somewhere like that. Molly was a big, strapping lass with jet black hair and the demeanour that 'encouraged' her fellow students to attend wholeheartedly. Even so, I found myself chatting to eight of her friends who were all keen to speak to the head of the CROUCHING community. In typical New York style they were loud, excitable and incredibly positive. They were also spreading the gospel to the various university campuses across the states and my 'You Tube' clips of various CROUCHES were being watched by thousands of kids all happy to 'go with it' as Molly always said. The recent Times Square CROUCH had been seen by over 35,000 people according to the 'You Tube' figures and even our recent noisy Peacocks CROUCH had now been viewed by nearly 15,000 people. After years of struggle, all of a sudden the CROUCHING community was beginning to flex its muscles and modern technology was helping me spread the word in ways I would once have never dreamed of. In Germany, Russia, Poland and particularly Latvia for some reason, community numbers had begun to rise sharply. Even down under in Australia and New Zealand images were being added to the website showing CROUCHES in all sorts of exotic venues, as well as lots of bars.

It was however, still in the U.K. where the CROUCHING community was strongest and most committed. It seemed inevitable that the number of members in America would soon overtake those here, but it was unlikely that anyone would match the home-grown CROUCHERS for sheer nuisance causing. I laughed loudly as I watched a video of the Liverpool end of the community go about picketing the Spar shop as promised and I counted thirty people all CROUCHING outside the entrance and holding a huge sheet which had the legend 'NO HAM WHAT A SHAM' painted across it. Apparently two of the community had been arrested and charged with public order offences which I found outrageous. It was just after five in the morning when I composed the following post:

The head of the CROUCHING community would like to offer a message of support to our friends and fellow members in Liverpool who boycotted their local Spar shop in response to another episode of ham related stock disaster. I understand that two people were arrested and subsequently charged by the Merseyside plod in what can only be described as a terrible ham related miscarriage of justice. I think I speak for the whole community in offering our support to our Liverpool members. I am considering what action to take and will keep you all posted as soon as a suitable act of retribution has been decided upon.

On a better note, our membership continues to grow rapidly and I would encourage everyone to encourage their friends, family and colleagues to CROUCH in random places as often as possible. I have found from experience that potential new members tend to enjoy the thrill of a CROUCH near a bus shelter or any pre – fabricated building. I aim to produce a list of random things to CROUCH next to which will help enhance the whole CROUCHING experience. A good starting point is near the gates of odd numbered bungalows especially if you know the owners to be elderly.

I am now off to lay face down on the kitchen floor to consider the problem of dead badger sniffing. I enjoy it, why doesn't anyone else?

Kirkland Christie   Head of the CROUCHING Community

Three hours later Gemma found me laying face down on the kitchen floor where I was still considering the most likely roads to find dead badgers on.

  "Have you been there all night?" She asked, stepping over me.

  "No, only since five," I answered slowly getting to my feet.

  "Oh right. Well that's okay then," she replied sarcastically, then added, "coffee?"

  "Please." I sat on one of the three kitchen stools and was silent as Gemma brewed the coffee. The percolator soon filled the kitchen with a lovely aroma and Gemma, for once in the morning, was in a really happy mood, enjoying the prospect of her two week break from work and the chance to spend time with the girls. When she was satisfied that the coffee was ready she poured us both a large mug and asked me what I had planned for the day.

  "I'm off for a quick CROUCH outside Hall, Graves and Lee, seeing as I missed it yesterday and then I'm hooking up with Craney and big Andy to sort out our outfits for Friday."

"So it's definitely happening then?"

"Of course it is," I answered quickly. "It's the U.K's first ever specialised round up of midgets. That reminds me; if I catch a couple can I put them in the garage?"

"Mate, if I come home and find a fucking midget in the garage I will go ape shit."

I nodded, understanding where she was coming from. "I know its dangerous Gem but the buggers will be tied up. They won't be able to get at you."

Gemma looked at me and shook her head. "You know mate, the worrying thing is that you're being completely serious. So let me make myself absolutely crystal fucking clear. No midgets in my garage."

"What about if I dig a pit at the bottom of the garden? Craney's already dug one in his."

"No, no fucking no."

We sat and talked for an hour, most of which was spent with me trying to persuade Gemma that bringing midgets home was a worthy, noble cause and Gemma responding by calling me a whole host of names in her delicate Manchester brogue. Eventually I gave up and went upstairs for a shower and by the time I was back downstairs the girls were up, watching some nonsense on T.V. and Gemma was busy smashing up the skirting boards with the hoover. I did my bit and hung out a load of washing and then headed off to the spiritual home of CROUCHING twenty four hours late but blessed by a beautiful spring morning. Although I had not had a wink of sleep I felt wide awake, enjoying the feel of the sunshine on my face and I fairly skipped along to my favourite CROUCHING spot.

It was ten past ten when Lucy rang me. I was in the middle of peering at a bush that ran alongside a low brick wall, considering whether it would make a good hiding place.

"Hello yes?"

"Hey you."

"I'm just doing a little hedge reconnaissance."

"I won't ask."

"You're calling early. You must be after my soft penis."

"You said it, Mr Softy." I heard her giggling.

"Have you found a way to increase your sex appeal yet woman?"

"I was thinking about covering my naked body in ham."

"Hang on; I thought I just felt a slight stirring."

"Twat. I'm just on my way to the hospital."

I had completely forgotten about her hospital appointment even though she had mentioned it a number of times the day before. "Are you worried?"

"Yes and no. I just want to get some answers. They probably won't tell me anything. It will just be more scans and more blood tests."

"Promise to call me as soon as you get out okay?"

"I promise. Right I'm nearly there, wish me luck."

"I'll be thinking of you fat head."

I left the hedge, in the end deciding it wasn't quite thick enough for really good hiding potential and twenty minutes later I was outside Hall, Graves and Lee performing a slick 140 degree left leg extension CROUCH, to the hoots of the workforce. As was always the case after a CROUCH outside the spiritual home of CROUCHING, I left feeling invigorated and walked the short distance to Craney's flat without stopping once to lean or check out any bushes. It was an ugly building on both the outside and the inside. Craney did however keep it clean and he was doing a pile of dishes as I walked in through the back door.

"Mr Christie, welcome to the palace of Craney." He waved a yellow rubber gloved hand in my direction.

"I can never get used to how domesticated you are mate," I said as he pulled off the gloves and left the few remaining unwashed dishes on the work top.

"I love a bit of cleaning matey. Sometimes I make a mess just so I can clean it up. Those dishes there," he motioned to the couple of plates he had left unwashed, "will get my attention when they least expect it."

"So what's with the day off anyway," I asked. "You didn't do a sicky for this did you?"

Craney shook his head. "The boss is in London. I've got a few bits to do later. Anyway, what's more important than sorting fancy dress out to go midget hunting in? I can't sleep with excitement." I believed him.

Craney was some sort of tree surgeon; that's what he called himself anyway. I think he just liked climbing things. That's probably why he got the job. He climbed the places no one else would do. He had offered to bring half a dozen chainsaws along to the hunt to 'worry the little fuckers' but after some serious consideration I had said no. I knew it would only end in disaster. The hunt was too important to me for that.

"They're in here," said Craney ushering me into the small lounge. There were half a dozen costumes hanging up on the sliding doors, Craney having a 'connection' at some party shop in town. "Yours is the one with the blue cover," he said pointing. I opened the cover and looked it over not intending to try it on but Craney was insistent and had already started stripping in order to show me his. I relented and five minutes later was admiring myself in the bathroom mirror and shouting downstairs to Craney that he had done me proud. I changed back and returned downstairs to find him running around the lounge in his costume like some demented madman.

"Let's go out now and see if we can get one. Try out the midget pit." He gestured to me to look out of the window to the small garden on the side of the house. Sure enough, there was a gaping hole right in the middle with a piece of wood adjacent to it with the words 'beware midgets' sprayed on it in bright yellow paint.

"I keep climbing in it to check it out for depth. I even asked my next door neighbour if I could borrow his eight year old daughter to see how she would manage. I think he reckons I'm some sort of kiddie fiddler now."

I laughed; Craney never did anything by halves. In fact he had another surprise for me.

"You know matey with the club foot?"

"What about him?"

"I got talking to him the other night, didn't I?" Craney had finally stopped running up and down the front room and turned to face me, a look of mischief in his eyes. "I was at John's two doors down having a smoke when who should bang at the door? It turns out he likes a smoke too. Anyway, getting to the point, I happened to have some very naughty skunk in my back pocket and it turns out that he has trouble getting it. So we did a deal. Let's just say you can expect a present on your door step tomorrow morning."

My heart skipped about six beats. "A big shoe?" I could hardly believe it.

"Freshly worn," said Craney proudly. I'm picking it up later. Apparently he has loads of them. I knew my prolific skunk smoking would pay dividends one day."

I clasped his hand and began to shake it. "What do you want in return mate?"

"Just look at it as a gift to the head of the CROUCHING community from its most loyal member."

"It's like a dream come true mate," I said honestly. And indeed it was. I had given up hope of ever owning one. Of course I could have probably gone on the internet and found one but that wasn't the same at all. This was a used one. The real deal so to speak. "I don't suppose you know what size it is?"

Craney shook his head. "No matey, but I'd be surprised if it fit you properly. He ain't very tall is he?"

I was just about to grill him further but my phone buzzed. In my excitement at Craney's news I had forgotten all about Lucy's hospital appointment. I almost even forgot to answer properly.

"Hello yes?"

"Hey."

"How did you get on?"

I heard a slight sigh down the phone. "More bloody tests. Just like I said would happen. I have to go back on Thursday."

"Surely they gave you some idea?" I was sure she was holding out on me.

"I don't know Kirk. They say one thing and then say something entirely different. I can't get my head around it. They want another scan and more blood. Fuck knows why they do. How much blood does it take for Christ's sake?" I could hear her voice cracking up. "I still don't have a clue what they're actually testing for."

"Didn't you ask?" I tried not to sound condescending.

"Of course I did." She snapped. Then said, "sorry, I'm just totally pissed off with it all."

"Hey, don't get upset fat head. There's nothing you can do until Thursday. Do you want to meet up?"

"I can't today Kirk. I've got to get back to work and I have a meeting at lunchtime."

"After work," I asked hopefully.

"Sorry, I can't. I've got a party to take the kids to. I'll be online later though."

"Okay fat head. Do you know I'm getting really soft talking to you?"

Lucy laughed loudly into my ear. "Twat!"

"That's right fat head, talk dirty to me. Make me softer!"

"Kirk, you really do cheer me up."

"And you fat head really do make me soft."

"Fuck off; you'll start giving me a complex."

"I think it must be your age," I went on. "I'm not used to getting into bed with woman over forty."

"You are surpassing yourself in twatishness today."

"Thanks. I'm at Craney's. He's only gone and got me a big shoe."

"A big shoe? Dare I ask?"

"He's dropping it around tomorrow morning. I'm over excited."

"Shame you weren't over excited yesterday."

"Yeah but this is a big shoe fat head."

"As opposed to my sexy body?"

"Exactly."

"I fucking give up with you. Right, I'm nearly back at work. Be online later and you can tell me all about your new shoe."

"Oh indeed I will."

We said our goodbyes and I went back into the front room to find Craney lying on the sofa, still in fancy dress. He pointed at the television and said, "I reckon I could become an antique dealer."

"Is this what you do on your days off? Watch shitty daytime T.V.?"

"Yep," he replied not looking up. "And wank." Then added, "vigorously."

I told him about my recent sexual 'non' encounter with Lucy.

"I'll get you some of that Viagra stuff matey. I don't think its actual Viagra but it's fucking brilliant. Jimmy at work was hard for three days."

I laughed, but was inherently cautious with anything Craney suggested was better than the real thing. I hoped that it wouldn't be long before my libido returned without the need for added assistance. "Right mate, get the kettle on." For the next couple of hours we discussed everything from the midget hunt to whether it was okay for Craney to shag his cousin. When I left we had agreed on everything that needed to be done before Good Friday and that it would be best if Craney went for a blow job off his cousin first and see how he felt after that before taking it any further.

I spent the rest of the day doing nothing much at all. I popped into the local library but gave up when about forty mothers and their babies came in. Far from being a peaceful retreat the place sounded worse than the Josh on a Saturday night. I walked to Larkham Lane and CROUCHED outside number 38 for five minutes and followed this by leaning on the telephone box in Underlane but to be honest I felt a bit lost hiking around the streets of Plympton without the sausage kings. Good Friday couldn't come quickly enough. I was feeling restless. Eventually I rang Nikki and walked over to hers for a glass of wine. Not long after I got there Gemma and the girls turned up and the three of us ended up drinking until nearly midnight. I was grilled about Lucy and had them in hysterics over the mister softy episode. I was more interested in raving about the big shoe but neither of them appeared in the slightest bit interested, such were they so used to my strange rants. Some people just didn't understand what was important in life. Give them a snippet of smut and they couldn't get enough.

We left just after midnight, with me insisting we walk the short journey rather than get a taxi. The girls were tired but excited about being out at night and this rose to fever pitch as they begged their mother to let me pinch another gate. Gemma was having none of it though, but I promised to bring them home a midget on Friday and that cheered them no end. When we got home I managed to persuade Gemma to have one last glass of wine before she went up to bed and soon after the house was silent and I was alone in front of the computer once more.

I opened up my Facebook page to find three messages from Lucy all saying 'where are you?' I looked at my watch which said ten past ten, shrugged and went to the CROUCHING in Random Places site. It had been a quieter day than of late and there was only a handful of new messages and two new photos. However, I was pleased to see one of the posts was from Mary Chang from the takeaway. It read:

Christie I hope you die fucking idiot soon.

Brilliant I thought. I found her Facebook page and made a post of my own:

The head of the CROUCHING community would like you to know Mary that no matter how much you beg. I cannot allow you to partake in next weekend's CROUCH outside Peacocks on The Ridgeway, Plympton. And no, I cannot be bribed with free chop suey.

I smiled and leaned back on the chair, almost tipping it back too far. Sometimes I found real pleasure in my work. My message should keep Mary fired up for a few more weeks. I was just about to make compose a message to Molly when Lucy appeared on my chat messenger thing, whatever you called it.

'At last!!!!'

'I've been drinking at Nikki's'

'I'm having a really shit time here....xxx'

'Excellent'

'Huge argument with old man'

'What about?'

'It doesn't matter but I can't stand much more of all the shit'

'Come over here for a bit of soft penis'

'Don't tempt me. I feel really down Kirk'

'I'm sorry fat head is there anything I can do?'

'Just carry on being you and make me smile'

'Well in just a few hours I shall hopefully be the proud owner of a big shoe. That's got to cheer you up'

'What is this big shoe thing anyway?'

'Check out club foot on Google'

'Ok. Two minutes'

I knew she'd take longer as she would use the excuse for a fag, so I went and made a cup of coffee. I took it back to the computer and waited for Lucy to come back. I bet she never thought she'd be searching the internet looking up club feet in the early hours of the morning.

'LOL you really are a twat Kirk'

'Just imagine the thrill of having a big shoe in your hands'

'I seriously think you've lost it. Absolutely barking you are'

'You wouldn't have me any other way'

'True. Love it! xxxxxx'

'I should hope so too. It takes a lot of practice to get this crazy'

'Right I have to get back to bed before he wonders what I'm doing. I really can't face another bust up!'

'Okay fat head xxx'

'I will call you in the morning xxxxxxxxxxxxxx'

'xxxxx'

With that she was gone and once more I was left alone to my own devices. I spent half an hour scouring the internet looking at images of people with a club foot. I was surprised to see how many varieties there were and apparently it was a fairly common disfigurement. Some of the big shoes were really quite fashionable these days which kind of ruined the whole thing. The big shoe had to be a straight forward black lace up with at least a three and a half inch raised sole. I was just mulling this over when Mary Chang messaged me again saying that she hoped I would die an agonising death, or some form of pidgin Chinese English to that effect. I was just about to reply to her when I heard my phone ping from the kitchen to say I'd received a text. I got up, wanting another coffee anyway and picking it up saw that it was from Craney. My heart raced.

'I am holding the big shoe in my hands' was all it said.

I smiled to myself and sent a message back. 'I never doubted your resolve mate. Treat yourself to an extra long spliff.' At last I thought. At last the big shoe was coming to me. The kettle boiled and as I poured the water into my mug, I could see my wide smile reflecting in the shiny chrome. It was distorted, which was probably about right. I went back to the computer and made one of the most pleasurable posts in a long time:

The head of the CROUCHING community has tonight had one of the best pieces of news in a very long time. Thank you Mr Crane, you never cease to amaze me. I am off to celebrate by having a late night aggressive ham eating session.

Kirkland Christie   Head of the CROUCHING Community

I was still on the computer, messaging members around the world when the girls came down and put the television on. I had been so engrossed in my work of spreading the CROUCHING gospel that I hadn't even noticed that it was light. Now, at the sight of the girls I suddenly realised that the big shoe should be sitting on the door step by now. Craney always started work early and would probably have left it before six o'clock. I checked my watch which said ten past ten and called out to the girls. "Go and see if someone has left a big shoe on the doorstep girls."

"A big shoe?" They both said at the same time.

"Yeah, a big shoe."

They didn't need any further encouragement and rushed off to the front door. I waited with bated breath and when I heard their squeals' of delight I knew Craney had done as he promised. They brought it in as if it were the crown jewels and held it up for me to admire. It was just as I had imagined. The huge black platform sole was scuffed and the laces frayed. It was a true original. I took it gently from the girls and held it up in front of me to look at properly. "It's magnificent," I said with a touch of awe in my voice.

"It's massive," said the girls.

I was still holding it up in front of me, deciding whether to wear it for my weekly appointment with the mental health nurse, when Gemma appeared in the doorway yawning, draped in a huge pink woolly dressing gown which dragged along the floor. I got up and held the big shoe in front of her face. "Gem, I want you to be the first one to sniff it." I turned the big shoe sideways so she could get her nose stuck in for a good sniff.

"What the fuck Kirk?" She said and pushed the shoe away. "What the hell is that?"

"It's a big shoe mum," shouted the girls. "It was on the doorstep."

"Club foot Gem," I said, as if that was meant to explain everything to her. "Craney got it for me. He left it outside on his way to work."

"I might have fucking guessed he'd have something to do with it. Wash your hands girls. God knows where it's been."

I put it down on the floor in front of me and attempted to slide my foot in. It was at least two sizes too small but that didn't stop me as I began to hobble lop sided up and down the front room. "Gem!" I shouted. "I'm wearing the big shoe!"

The girls came back in after washing their hands and began to march up and down beside me and then began to argue about who was going to try it on next. Gemma eventually lost her rag and screamed at the lot of us to "shut the fuck up." I don't think the fact that she had a hangover was helping her see the big shoe in the best of lights. I took her subtle hint and disappeared upstairs for a shower, leaving the girls to take the brunt of her bad temper. I placed the big shoe on my small bedside chest of drawers and couldn't help coming back into the bedroom twice to look at it before getting into the shower.

As far as I could tell I hadn't had a wink of sleep in the last two nights yet I didn't feel particularly tired. Even so the shower felt good, for the nothing else than to prepare me mentally for the day ahead; a day where I was now the owner of a big shoe. I wondered how much owning it would change me. I was trying to make my mind up when Lucy rang me on her way to work. Before I could mention the big shoe she blurted out that she couldn't talk but wanted to come and see me straight after work and that it was important. I said of course and was trying to get the words 'big shoe' out when she said she had to go and ended the call. It was a most strange one way conversation which left me deflated after my earlier excitement. Something was up, there had been a real sense of urgency in her voice and it worried me no end. I didn't know what I'd do if something went wrong with our burgeoning relationship.

I spent twenty minutes admiring the big shoe before heading off to my parents for yet another mental health session, this time my regular weekly one with my CPN; community psychiatric nurse. I walked briskly, trying not to worry about Lucy. I had become incredibly attached to her and shared all my inner most thoughts (however strange) with her. She on the other hand held an awful lot back, as the recent heart problem showed and although we agreed to be open with each other I knew she kept a lot of stuff from me. Whether this was to protect me or for other reasons I had no idea but up to this point I had never felt even the tiniest bit concerned about our relationship. Now as I walked along the quiet streets, I racked my brain for reasons why she was suddenly making such urgent demands. It was impossible though. It could be anything from her health to her husband. In the end I gave up and hid in one of the large laurel bushes next to the path at Harewood House. As usual I starting barking and had to call it a day after ten minutes when two real dogs started barking back at me.

It somewhat surprised me that I talked openly about Lucy to the CPN. In fact I talked of little else throughout the thirty minute meeting. I handily left out her marital status or that I had packed in taking my medication so I could hopefully have sex at some point soon. I did say though that she was the best thing that had happened to me since my marriage had ended and that I was finally feeling like I could embrace normal society again. All in all it wasn't a bad meeting but if anything I was just reaffirming to myself how important she was to me.

My parents seemed happy that I seemed to be behaving myself although I did have to answer a thousand questions from my mother about 'this new woman' in my life. After a lunch of tomato soup and cheese sandwiches I made my way back to Gemma's resisting all urges to deviate on the way. Besides, I was anxious to get back to the big shoe. The house was empty and I rushed up to my bedroom to check on the big shoe. It was just where I left it although it had the addition of a piece of paper sticking out of the inside. I grabbed the paper and saw that it was a note from Gemma. All it said was, 'NUTTER' along with some kisses. I smiled and picked up the big shoe and once more admired its undeniable beauty. For the rest of the afternoon I walked around the house wearing it and talked to myself about everything from the midget problem to whether it would be possible to set fire to the neighbour's garden shed and get away with it. When the doorbell rang I was surprised at where the afternoon had gone. I checked my watch; it said ten past ten. I took off the big shoe and went to the front door.

Lucy looked amazing and for the second time that day I felt my heart skip a few beats, although not quite as many as when I first held the big shoe. I ushered her inside and she went swiftly past me to the kitchen saying, "I'm in desperate need of a glass of wine Kirk."

I followed her in and had the big shoe held up in front of her as she turned from the fridge with a bottle of unopened white chardonnay in her hand.

"Look at it fat head," I said excitedly. "Look at the sheer beauty of it."

Lucy shook her head and said, "It's beautiful Kirk, now where are the glasses?"

I grabbed a couple off the draining board and waited as she unscrewed the top and poured us both a healthy measure. Gemma insisted on buying screw top and not corked bottles and it was a constant bone of contention. Lucy took a large mouthful and let out a long sigh, then lit a cigarette. I left my glass on the work top and held the big shoe in front of her. "You can sniff the inside if you want. It's a proper used one."

"That's disgusting," Lucy replied between rapid puffs on the cigarette.

"I beg your pardon fat head. It's the nicest thing I have ever offered you. Look at the size of it woman." My enthusiasm for once didn't seem to be having the desired effect. When

Lucy didn't even smile at my suggestion I asked her, "so come on fat head, what's up? Something's bugging you. Do you want to wear the big shoe in private for a while? I can go upstairs if it helps."

All of a sudden tears began to roll down her cheeks and for once I was a little lost for words. She reached out and put her hands into mine and I got a nervous feeling in the pit of my stomach.

"Right, there's no easy way to say this, my old man has booked us a surprise trip to France next week. My sister's having the kids and my parents are giving us their Jag to travel in. They all think it will be great for me given the health stuff and the relationship problems." Her words came out in a torrent; no doubt she had rehearsed this little speech all day. I said nothing but just stood and waited. She took a gulp of wine and went on, "It may well be the case I end up having an operation and they all thought it would be nice to have a quiet break in the meantime." I still said nothing so she offered, "I found out last night but I didn't want to tell you on the computer. I've been shitting myself all day. Kirk," she shook my arms, "I don't want to go. I really don't."

After another few awkward seconds I finally said something. "Then don't go. You're a big girl. Just say no."

"I wish it was that easy Kirk. My sister has taken a week off work, mother has rang my boss to get special permission for the time off and everything has been paid for."

"I don't know what to say." I actually didn't. "I'm going to miss you. An awful lot. When do you go?"

"Sunday." She couldn't look me in the eye.

"Wow. Everyone's leaving me. Did you know Gemma is going to Penzance with her sister for the Easter weekend?"

"I'm so sorry Kirk. I really am."

I picked up the big shoe and looked at it sadly. My perfect day was rapidly going downhill.

"I really don't want to spend even a second apart from you Kirk."

"Really?" My question was loaded with sarcasm.

"Really." She came over to me and I let her take the big shoe from me and put it down on the work surface. She wrapped her arms around me and reached up, pulling my head down to meet her. Her soft lips pushed against mine and I could taste the salt of her tears on them as we kissed. Her eyes were closed but I looked down over her shoulder at the big shoe and little by little I felt a slow stirring in my groin. Either the medication was leaving my bloodstream or the big shoe was arousing me in ways Lucy could only dream of. When she finally released me from her vice like grip she said softly, "want to have another try Mr Softy?

"If you wear the big shoe in bed I'll fuck you senseless." I half meant it.

"Twat." She took my hand and pulled me towards the staircase. I had picked up the big shoe and was clinging to it tightly as I let Lucy lead me up the stairs. When we reached the top she let go of me saying, "get into bed," and darted into the bathroom. I carefully placed the big shoe on the chest of drawers next to the bed and stripped naked, sprayed some Armani, a lot more carefully this time and slid under the duvet. I reached down to my crotch and fiddled around a bit. There was definitely something happening. I was still fiddling around when Lucy came in. For the second time that day I couldn't believe my luck.

"You like?" She said as I took in the view of her in a black basque and stockings along with her dangerously high stilettos. "I thought this might help Mr Softy?"

She looked incredibly sexy and instantly took my mind off her upcoming vacation. At long last after God knows how long Kirkland Christie, the head of the CROUCHING community had something approaching an erection. Lucy yanked the quilt back and smiled greedily as she saw that she had achieved the desired effect. She kissed me briefly on the cheek and said, "enjoy," and slipped down to take me in her mouth. I laid back with my hands behind my back and tried to concentrate on the matter in hand. Already the spectre of Uncle Percy was hovering somewhere close by.

Lucy eventually finished with her coxing of my cock and came up to kiss me and then quickly slid onto my erection, gasping and squealing with delight at the same time. She sat straight up and began to slowly ride me, her eyes closed as she lost herself in the moment. After a couple of minutes she began to twist and pinch her nipples and I stretched up to join in, licking and biting them. "Fucking harder," she moaned pulling my head into her breasts. I winced at the pressure my teeth must have been exerting on her but she just moaned ever louder and instructed me politely to, "fucking bite my fucking nipples." A few seconds later came the words that all men like to hear. "I'm fucking coming!" I hoped Gemma didn't suddenly walk in the front door. Mind you, the window was slightly open and Lucy's lustful roar would probably upset the neighbours for months. Finally she calmed, her climax had been brief but fierce and she bent down and kissed me passionately. "Now it's your turn big boy." She slid back off me and once again went downstairs and slurped greedily on my cock. She demanded that I come in her mouth which was fine by me. The good thing about Lucy being down below so to speak was that she couldn't see me silently mouthing the words, "mercy mercy Uncle Percy" over and over again. I was getting to the point of no return and if I was being honest I was more fearful than lustful.

Lucy could obviously sense that things were coming to a head and really went to work on me; her greedy slurping sounds and murmured urgings only bringing about the inevitable climatic disaster which I now couldn't hope to prevent.

"Come in my mouth," was the last thing I remember clearly and come in her mouth I did.

"MERCY MERCY UNCLE PERCY!"

My words came out like a thunderbolt. I shouted like I was at a football match. Lucy began to splutter and cough violently at the shock of my vocal announcement. She sat up, her eyes watering, trying to catch her breath and with one huge retching sound spluttered a healthy amount of my warm love juice into my face. She then scrambled off the bed and rushed into the bathroom sounding like she was choking to death. I lay motionless, my one clear eye looking at the big shoe. "Fucking Uncles," I said quietly and reached for a towel that was hung over the radiator. I did my best to wipe my face clean and was still at it when Lucy came back into the bedroom, her face and her eyes red.

"Alright fat head?" I said cheerily.

"What the fuck was that all about?" She replied, less cheerily.

"What do you mean?"

"Uncle fucking Percy, what do you think?"

"I thought that's what all blokes shouted when they come."

Lucy stood at the bottom of the bed staring at me in disbelief. "You never cease to amaze me," she said shaking her head. I was thinking how hot she still looked.

"I know. I'm glad you enjoyed it so much."

"I'm literally speechless," was all she could say back.

I crawled forward on the bed towards her and grabbed her hand. "I'm sure Uncle Percy is very proud of you fat head."

Lucy tried to be angry but just couldn't keep herself from bursting out laughing. "Fucking hell you're mad Kirk. I can't believe you sometimes." She climbed back onto the bed minus the stilettos and curled up against me, her head resting on my chest. I stroked her hair and said quietly, "do you really have to go away?"

"Don't Kirk," she replied. "Please don't make a big deal about it. It's not even a week. I'll be back before you know it."

"I'm going to really miss you." I meant it.

"I'll miss you more, believe me baby." She raised her head to kiss me. "I intend to spend as much time with you as I possibly can before I go."

"Lots of rude stuff?" I asked.

"An awful lot of very rude stuff."

"You know you could come on the midget hunt to make up for leaving me."

"I don't think so," Lucy laughed loudly. "Anyway I'm doing my best to make sure I can get the evening off to spend with you."

"I suppose you're hoping I return from the hunt feeling all manly and stud like."

She laughed again. "Yeah, something like that."

I stroked her hair again and asked her if there was anything more she was holding back on me about her heart problem.

For a while she was quiet, I guessed she was thinking about what to tell me. Eventually she said, "It doesn't sound good. They told me there was a chance I was suffering from premature ventricular contractions. I think that's what the consultant called it. It's all to do with my heart skipping a beat. I had a load more blood taken to see if I have an electrolyte imbalance or something. Whatever the hell that means. If I have it then It's apparently quite nasty. If I don't then it's not too serious at all."

"You probably need one of those sports drinks. The ones that replace electrolytes."

"Twat."

"Seriously though fat head, how do you feel about it all?"

She thought for a moment and answered probably truthfully, "as always I'm just burying my head, the same as I always do."

"When you say serious, how serious?"

"I'm not even thinking about it until I know for sure."

"Okay sweetheart, I mean fat head. Just promise to be honest with me however tough things turn out to be."

"I promise." She reached up and kissed me again and we clung to each other, two souls lost in their problematic worlds, Lucy worrying about her impending test results and whether she would need a heart operation, me wondering when I could next walk around in the big shoe. Eventually Lucy sat up, "Kirk, I best be going, I'm late as it is."

"I was hoping you'd hang around for another eight hours or so. I might be ready for another go by then."

"You never know, I may find time tomorrow lunchtime if you have an empty house."

"Believe me the house will be empty, even if I have to lock Gemma and the girls in the garage."

"Good. I may even wear my black stockings again if you're lucky," Lucy said with a mischievous grin.

"And I may wear the big shoe if you're lucky," I responded.

"And with that image in my head I need to get myself sorted." She got up off the bed much to my protestations, grabbed her clothes and went into the bathroom to change. I remained in bed looking at the big shoe again and marvelling at its magnificent sole. Lucy caught me staring at it when she reappeared looking not the least bit like she'd been fucking my brains out less than half an hour ago. "I can see I'm going to have problems with you and that shoe. Right Uncle Percy, I'm off. I will see you tomorrow." She blew me a kiss, not trusting me enough to bend down to kiss me and a minute later I heard her car pull away outside. I stared at the big shoe for another ten minutes before finally getting up myself and heading for the shower. I stayed under the hot water for a long time, finally letting the news of Lucy's imminent departure to France sink in. Everyone was leaving me. When I finally turned off the water I could hear that Gemma and the girls had returned home. I pulled on a tracksuit and made my way downstairs, my hair still wet.

"Nikki is coming over for pizza. Iceland had a two for one offer," she told me, knowing I wasn't the least bit interested in Iceland and it's two for one offers.

I smiled and grabbed a beer from the fridge. I made no mention of the afternoon's shenanigans; that could wait until Nikki had arrived.

CHAPTER ELEVEN

DO YOU HAVE SEX ANALLY OR MORE THAN ONCE A YEAR?

CROUCHING Community Membership 4,233

I don't know who laughed most although Gemma did have to rush to the toilet saying she was about to wet herself. When the kids came into the kitchen to ask what was so funny, Nikki told them that I had been to visit my Uncle Percy and then started crying with laughter again. Gemma came back in saying she had had to change her knickers.

"I knew I'd get your knickers down eventually," I said smiling.

"I'm worried I'm going to shout it out now the next time I have sex," cried Nikki, tears rolling down her cheeks.

"It's addictive Nikki. Once it's in your head you have to shout it out."

"You better make sure you keep your fucking window shut in future Kirk," Gemma said seriously. "I've got enough trouble with the neighbours with your bloody sign collecting."

The conversation carried on like this for the rest of the evening and when Nikki and her daughters left and Gemma had shooed hers up to bed the house was suddenly very quiet. I topped up Gemma's glass and she asked, "so how do you feel about Lucy going away then?"

"What can I do Gem? She's married. I'm obviously not happy about it and I'm going to miss her like mad. It doesn't help with Zak being away and the sausage kings," I moaned.

"Are you going to be okay with us going to Cornwall? I feel really bad about it now. I can easily cancel it mate."

Gemma was so lovely I thought to myself. I knew she meant it. "I'll be fine Gem. And you've been looking forward to a bit of a break."

"Nikki's going to keep an eye on you and make sure you're okay. And I'm going to be ringing constantly. You'll probably be totally pissed off with us both by the time I get back."

Gemma was taking the girls to some caravan park near Penzance with her sister. It would be the first time I had been left on my own for any significant period of time. Thank God I had the big shoe to keep me company I thought.

"Are you worried this France thing will bring her and her husband closer together mate? I hate to say it but it might you know." She reached out and squeezed my hand.

"I really don't know Gem. Probably, knowing my luck. It's fucking typical, just as things are going well. I'm wondering whether she's known about the holiday for ages and just didn't tell me until it was right on top of her."

"Listen mate, you may well find that it's a disaster and ends up being the final straw for them. If she's as crazy about you as she appears to be, then a few days away isn't going to change a thing."

"I don't think I'm strong enough for another emotional disaster Gem." I meant it.

"Well don't go beating yourself up over it every day she's away. There's nothing you can do but wait until she's back. And she will be back mate."

"It's going to be a very long week," I went on, taking a sip of awful tasting 'Gemma special' cheap wine. "I can already envisage a lot of hedges being hidden in around Plympton."

"And no doubt a lot of kitchen lino sniffing," Gemma added laughing. "See, there's plenty of constructive things to do with your time."

"I'll probably spend the week down Craney's guarding the midget pit. You know, feeding them and poking them with sticks, that sort of thing."

Gemma put her head in her hands. "The problem is I believe you. I can see I'm going to have to ring you every twenty minutes not every hour." She drained the last of her drink and added, "right I'm going up and you need to get some sleep too."

She was right of course. "Yeah I know. I just need to check a couple of things and then I'll be up too."

Twenty minutes later I was still reading all the latest messages and hadn't even started with the e mails when Lucy butted in on my work.

'Hey you xxx'

'Hello fat head xx'

'I'm feeling really horny'

'Are you?'

'Yeah big time'

'Well you have less than 12 hours to wait'

'I know!!!!!!!!!'

'Tell me something, do you have sex anally or more than once a year?'

'I know there's a catch here'

'Well???'

'Basically you want to know if I like bottom sex.'

'Or I could be asking if you like sex more than once a year.'

'The answer is yes'

'To which one?'

'Ha ha ha'

'Dirty girl'

'Very x'

'I'm gutted about next week'

'Me too'

'What if you fall back in love with your old man?'

'LOL. It's not going to happen'

'Stranger things have happened. Take the big shoe. Who would have thought a few days ago that I would have had one in my hands?'

'Kirk, it is NOT going to happen xxx'

'Promise?'

'PROMISE xxxxx'

'The next 48 hours are going to be incredible'

'???'

'Well anal sex with you tomorrow and the midget hunt on Friday'

'LOL I may have been saying I only have sex once a year'

'Shit! Typical'

'I trust there will be no sign of Uncle Percy?'

'One can never tell when Uncle Percy may arrive'

'I'll have to gag you'

'Interesting...'

'Kinky...'

'I always thought you'd turn out to be a pervert fat head'

'Anything to get shot of Uncle Percy'

'I'll remember that and put it to good use'

'Involving ham and the big shoe by any chance?'

'More than likely'

'Twat'

'You have to ring the hospital tomorrow don't you? Or should I say later today?' I looked at my watch. It said ten past ten.

'Yep, can't wait. Shitting it!!'

'I bet. But whatever the outcome I promise to take your mind off it at lunchtime'

'I'm counting on it. I'm going to be VERY hungry at lunchtime you know'

'You really are quite bad fat head'

'Not quite – very!'

'Can't wait'

'I'll be starving xxxx'

'Will you please stop it? I don't want you making me soft before I go to bed.'

'Twat. Right on that note I'm off to bed. I need my beauty sleep.'

'Okay fat head. Have dirty dreams about me xxx'

'Always xxx'

I could definitely feel stirrings in my crotch now and for the thousandth time wondered what such a beautiful and sexy woman saw in me, a social pariah. Mind you a social pariah who was the head of Europe's largest knee bending concern, I might add.

Putting all thoughts of lust to one side I got on with the job in hand, my late night Trans – Atlantic CROUCHING gospel sermons. Tonight I found myself in conversation with a couple of guys in El Paso, Texas. I imagined crowds of cowboys in chaps and spurs climbing from their horses to CROUCH in dusty deserts. No doubt it was nothing like this whatsoever but it was a nice thought and I loved the fact that the CROUCHING community had now reached the Lone Star state. I was also rewarded with a terrific photo from Philadelphia of half a dozen school kids CROUCHING on the roof of their yellow school bus. I didn't catch up with Molly but it was incredible how things were developing across the pond. I spent a further thirty minutes answering various questions before making the following post:

It is less than 48 hours until the inaugural Good Friday Midget Hunt. I know that for many of you the nerves must be jangling and the urge to hunt overwhelming. We must however, restrain ourselves until the official start of the hunt as any attempt to tackle a midget alone will not only lead to failure but is also highly dangerous, as I have recently found out to my own cost. Under NO circumstances should anyone ever attempt to secure a midget without sufficient back up no matter how much it taunts you. I would go as far as saying that a large headed variety would need at least half a dozen hunters to get it under control. I know that we are all sick of the stupid 'red tape' health and safety nonsense that Brussels' bombards us with, but in this matter I really cannot stress enough the need for caution.

In regard to all the photos I have been sent of kid's heads from worried parents, I can categorically state that as of all the ones I have seen up to today, there is none that appear to be oversized or have water melon like features. I do urge though, to continue to measure your children's heads on a regular basis.

Kirkland Christie   Head of the CROUCHING Community

Seconds after making the post I was delighted to see Mary Chang's name pop up on my screen.

'I see you now upset midget idiot prick'

'Not upsetting them Mary, hunting them.'

'You are fucking idiot prick'

'And you are yellow'

'Fucking racit pig'

'I'm considering CROUCHING outside your takeaway again'

'You do I fuck kill you'

'Excellent, I look forward to it Mary'

'You are prick fucking pig idiot'

'Tell me Mary, do you measure your children's heads?'

'My children grown up fuck idiot'

'Ah, so at least you are aware of what I am talking about. I am glad to see you read all my posts and take my messages seriously. Did you bandage their feet when they were young?

'Fuck off idiot I kill you'

'By food poisoning?'

'Fuck off and die you come here I fuck dead you are'

'I haven't got a clue what you are on about Mary but just promise me you won't try to force feed me'

'Ass fuck licker'

And on that Shakespearean note the wonderfully angry Mary Chang was gone. I wondered how much she truly hated me. Probably quite a lot. I went to my Twitter account and tweeted: 'I have been called, racist, a prick, an idiot and better off dead. I am pleased my ban of the Chinese from CROUCHING is being taken so well.'

I was about to switch off the computer and hit the hay for some much needed shut eye when I suddenly decided to make one final post:

Recently the head of the CROUCHING community has been blessed by a beautiful woman entering my life. This has forced me to ask difficult questions of myself, things that I have avoided for many years, such as: is unsmoked ham better than smoked? Does wafer thin stack up against a standard cut? All I can say is that any ham is better than no ham at all.

Kirkland Christie   Head of the CROUCHING Community

When I woke up the following morning I felt groggy; my body was in need of at least another eight hours of shut eye. However, I was pleased to have managed any sleep at all considering I had stopped my medication. I had visions of being awake for a week. My dreams however had been terrible. Dreams within dreams I called them. I always suffered when I stopped taking the Venlafaxine for more than a couple of days. I would have a nightmare and wake up dripping in sweat and then some faceless creature would jump out from under my bed and attack me and then I'd wake up again. It went on like this all night and was truly frightening. My bed was drenched with sweat and would definitely need changing before Lucy arrived. I sniffed it to make sure that's all it was soaked with. For the rest of the morning I relived my dreams as if they were real, forming memories in my head that were all pervading and pushed all my other ones aside. In other words it was like my dreams were absolutely real and had happened.

I had badgered Gemma the night before about disappearing for a couple of hours over lunchtime and she had reluctantly taken the girls off to the cinema. In return she had made me promise to get rid of all the For Sale signs and the gate. It was a lot easier than I thought it would be as all I had to do was throw it all on the garage roof. It took less than ten minutes. I was pacing up and down the front room with the big shoe on when the door bell rang. Lucy had arrived.

I ushered her in and once again she looked fantastic. Her skirt was shorter than before and she was again wearing stockings and high heels just like the day before. She immediately wrapped her arms around me and gave me a long passionate kiss. "Get upstairs," I ordered and gave her a slap on the arse which made her squeal with delight.

"Don't I even get a drink," Lucy said as I pushed her up the stairs.

"Later," I replied. "You have to earn it." I had changed from someone not a bit interested in sex for three years into some raging nymphomaniac in a few short days. This time she didn't even make the bathroom; I pushed her straight into the bedroom and flung her onto the bed. She rolled over laughing and looked up at me, pulled me to her, gave me a naughty look and unbuttoned my jeans. This time my cock needed no extra encouragement to stand tall and fairly burst out of my boxers and into Lucy's welcoming mouth. She needed no encouragement and greedily went to work on me, her eyes looking up at mine as she did a good job of imitating some American porn star. This time though I stopped her well before it went too far, so to speak and pulling on her hair I finally got her to leave my cock alone long enough to allow me to strip. Lucy got the hint and began to remove her work gear. However, I wasn't expecting to be greeted by the sight of an incredibly sexy black basque, so tight her large boobs were only just managing to not burst out.

"You like?" Lucy purred twanging one on the suspenders holding up a fancy topped black stocking.

"It's okay," I replied, "but I'm more of a woolly vest sort of guy."

"Twat. I'll have to leave it here though. You can put it next to the big shoe while I'm away to remind you of me." She pulled down onto the bed and them immediately rolled over and climbed on top of me. She began to slowly tease me, I could feel my erection rubbing around her tiny black g string which was begging to be ripped off, but when I made a grab for it she slapped my hand and said, "not yet baby." She kissed me again, biting at my tongue and then murmured a little breathlessly, "suck my tits. Hard." She pulled my head hard into her cleavage and without much encouragement her big tits burst out of the basque and I did exactly as I was told. This time I didn't hold back and I roughly bit Lucy's nipples which made her gasp and swear in equal measure. When she could take no more she slid back down and went to work on my cock again. I pulled on her hair so hard I was expecting a clump to come out in my hand but Lucy seemed to love it. I tried not to think of the woman from the Home Prevention Team and her alopecia but the image lodged itself in my head so I lifted her back up and told her to fuck me.

"How about you fuck me?" Lucy said and rolled over onto her stomach. I needed no further encouragement and knelt over her, pulling her up onto all fours. She let out a long moan of pleasure as I roughly entered and went about the business of 'fucking her brains out'. Whereas I was quiet and focused, Lucy shouted expletives and demanded I pull her hair. I had made a point of closing my window before she arrived but I still reckoned half the street would be able to hear her. After a few minutes of pounding I let go of her hair and moved my attention to her wonderful arse. I gave it a few hard slaps much to Lucy's pleasure, who predictably shouted, "fucking harder," but I ignored her this time and instead concentrated on the anal sex angle. I allowed my fingers to gently rub her arsehole, softly caressing her trying to get a hint if this was out of bounds. Lucy's demeanour didn't change so I gave my middle finger a quick lick and slid it slowly into her. This time she offered a low moan but said nothing to discourage me; if anything she just pushed on me harder. This was all the encouragement I needed so I desperately began looking around for something to act as a lubricant. My eyes finally settled on a pot of a hair gel which at the push I should just be able to reach. I grabbed Lucy's hair with one hand and made a lunge with the other and just managed to grab the pot before Lucy really would resemble the woman from the Home Prevention Team. Fortunately she just thought I was being rough with her and moaned a tad louder if that was possible. I quickly removed the lid and took a huge handful of the red slippery gel and slapped it around her arsehole. Lucy baulked at the sudden shock of the cold substance and pulled away causing me to slip out of her. "What the fuck's that?" She uttered reaching a hand around to feel it.

"Your arse needs to be abused woman."

"You reckon?" Lucy said breathlessly but made no attempt to stop me.

With my cock already free I rubbed a load more hair gel over it and pushed it up against Lucy's anus. She let out a grunt followed by, "you dirty fucker," followed by a cry of "fucking yes!" as I slid my way into her most private of parts. You couldn't describe this as love making, it was far from it. This was pure dirty and aggressive sex. I went at her hammer and tong and she shouted both encouragement and abuse at me repeatedly. We fucked like our lives depended on it and after years of neglect my cock was finally getting the outing it had been waiting for. When I was finally about to climax there had not been one thought of Uncle Percy or Mr Softy. I slid myself out of her and she instantly rolled over to face me and demanded that I come over her tits. I just made it in time and for once nothing went wrong. I covered her wonderfully large breasts in my seamen (to put it politely) as Lucy told me to "let it all out baby." When I was spent she pulled me down to her and kissed me and we lay inseparable in my sticky mess.

"You're so gorgeous Lucy," I said quietly. "I can't believe how sexy you are."

"Fucking hell!" Lucy barked. "You called me Lucy!"

"It must be love."

"Lust more like," she said laughing.

"I cannot believe what you've just made me do," I said with a serious tone.

"Twat," Lucy responded still laughing.

"Yuck," I peeled myself off of her. "Do you fancy sharing a shower?"

"Definitely," she replied making a face at all the mess over her.

We got up and went into the bathroom; Lucy kicking off her shoes and undoing her stockings, having to grab hold of me to stop her falling over as she did so.

"You may as well keep the basque on, you know; give it a bit of a wash. It certainly needs it."

Lucy laughed, yanked her g string off and climbed into the shower cubicle with me, still looking sexy as hell although a lot shorter. She quickly began to wash the front of her basque "I can't believe you've forced me to wear it in the shower."

"And I can't believe you forced me into having anal sex with you."

She kissed me, the water running into my mouth as she did. "You are an extremely naughty man Kirk Christie." Then added, "do not get my hair wet on pain of death."

"You should be more concerned with how short you are without your shoes. I really am considering measuring your head."

"And locking me in your garage?"

"Definitely. And keeping you as my sex slave."

"Maybe you ought to get a tape measure then." She laughed and reached up and kissed me passionately. As I kissed her back, the water pouring over my head as Lucy pulled her hair to safety I felt her hand slowly begin to massage me down below and much to my amazement my old boy began to react. "Hello, somebody wants seconds." Lucy began to stroke me more quickly.

"It's the power of the big shoe," I said and reached down and lifted her small body up unto me. She wrapped her legs tightly around me, her back pressed against the cubicle wall. There was no biting, hair pulling or swearing second time around. Instead we kissed each other passionately as I slowly moved inside her; Lucy gyrating her hips gently. We looked into each other's eyes with an understanding born out of need; no words would have sufficed. Yet as I looked into her pale blue eyes I could still see some deep seated sadness that I couldn't quite fathom. As we both came close to climax, Lucy's gyrations sped up and she broke free of our kiss and whispered in my ear, "I love you Kirk, I really do love you."

"And I love you too fat headed one," I said back a second before I came. I was going to say Lucy but once in a day was enough. I didn't want her getting the wrong impression. Mind you, I must admit it was one of the better showers I had had in recent years.

After a few more minutes Lucy finally removed the basque and gave herself a quick wash down, doing everything to keep her hair from getting wet, whilst I went about splashing her, doing everything I could to get it wet. After plenty of expletives she finally managed to get out of the cubicle and wrote 'TWAT' in huge letters in the condensation on the shower door. It actually said 'TAWT' but I didn't have the heart to tell her. By the time I had washed myself and got out of the shower Lucy had disappeared back into the bedroom to dress. I wandered in still naked and found her fussing over her hair in the mirror. Unlike our previous encounters her hair was tousled and her cheeks bright red. I pointed it out, "unlike last time you look properly fucked today."

"Unlike last time, today I have been."

"Oi watch it pervert."

She pulled on her shoes, suddenly gaining many inches and came over to me and put her arms around my neck. "I don't have to stand on tip toe again now."

"You would if I wasn't bending down."

She tutted. "I really wish I was taller."

"Get away," I smiled. "You're cute."

"Cute?"

"Very cute."

"Twat. Right I really need to go Kirk."

We kissed briefly this time and I pulled on a pair of boxers and followed her down the stairs to the front door.

"Don't go leaving my basque lying around for Gemma to find, Kirk."

"Don't worry fat head, I won't be taking it off."

She shook her head and ran up the steps, shouting over her shoulder before she reached her car, "The worrying thing is I believe you."

I watched her drive quickly off and was just about to close the door when I saw the next door neighbour staring at me; she was holding a pair of pruning shears and had been pretending to do a bit of gardening but really had been listening to us. I smiled at her and said loudly, "prostitute. She caters for all types of needs." I closed the door and went upstairs to clear up. The bedroom looked like a bomb had hit it and the bathroom was half flooded. It took a good twenty minutes to get it looking something like Gemma kept it and I had just started on my bedroom when my phone buzzed on the chest of drawers next to the big shoe. It was a text from Lucy saying, 'my bum hurts.' I replied, 'my willy smells' to which the inevitable, 'twat' response came instantly back.

I tidied the room quickly, dressed and went down to the kitchen and made myself a ham sandwich. I grabbed an ice cold bottle of beer and went into to the dining room and sat down in front of the PC. I made just one tweet: 'you can run and you can hide but sooner or later we're gonna track you down. 24 hours to go.'

I decided I needed a bit of fresh air to clear the fug which had returned now that Lucy had gone, so I switched off the computer and went out for a walk. I wanted a bit of clear headed thinking time before the following day's festivities so I even left my earphones behind. I headed off in no particular direction unable to concentrate for the time being as all I could think about was the incredible sex I had just had. The images rolled across my mind like a porn film with me and Lucy as the stars. She had even told me she loved me. Did she mean it or was she just saying it in the heat of the moment? What would she be thinking after a week away with her husband? Was she as sexy in bed with him? Was she on the pill? Was she measuring her children's heads regularly? There were so many things to worry about. With all these thoughts and many more like them, I gave up trying to think about the midget hunt and decided to ring all the main protagonists instead. I spoke to Big Andy who confirmed what Craney had said about picking me up in the Transit just before eleven. Craney himself just shouted, "I am the midget master" down the line and hung up. I left messages with a number of other hunters and after a couple of attempts got hold of Lenny who said his camera and tablet were all ready to go. The tablet would be used to keep abreast with all midget activity and potential sightings. When Carter rang me back shouting something about wanking to midget porn last night I knew we were all good to go.

I was close to St Mary's Church so I decided to go inside and see the vicar. We had become acquainted over the last few years as I would often wander in and sit down on a pew waiting for some sort of divine intervention to change my life. Usually these related to new places to CROUCH outside. For once the church was reasonably busy, by that I mean there was more than three people inside its vast emptiness. I remembered it was Easter week and tried to think what today was. Maundy Thursday? I should know considering I sang here as a choir boy for three years many moons ago. I sat down on a pew just inside the side entrance and looked around for the vicar but saw no sign of him. As usual I found myself wishing it was a Catholic place of worship which had one of those confession boxes in it. I could have confessed to all sorts of things like painting the words 'flying cunts' in bright red paint outside Ken's Birds shop or for when I put a dead badger on the middle of the bowling green at Harewood House. I wondered if I would have the nerve to tell a priest that I had just fucked a married woman up the harris? I probably shouldn't be thinking such thoughts in church so I tried to put Lucy out of my mind and focus on the midget hunt.

After about ten minutes the vicar appeared at the back of the church. Or was it the front? Or the East? I got up and made my way towards him, treading in the same footsteps that my parents had forty five years before on their wedding day. I called out to the vicar who turned and greeted me amiably. "Hello Kirkland. What brings you to St Mary's then? Have you run out of places to CROUCH?"

"There are always places that need CROUCHING outside of vicar, including your church."

"I'm sure we'd be most honoured," he replied.

"One Sunday I will bring the community down here and you can CROUCH with us vicar. You may even have an epiphany."

"Quite," the vicar said not really knowing how to answer such a statement.

"Have you got a minute vicar? I wanted to ask your advice on something."

The elderly man smiled at me benignly, placed the folder he was carrying down on a pew and gestured me to sit. "Of course my son; as long as it's not about the Chinese again."

A few months ago I had claimed to have seen a number of suspicious looking Chinese men on the church roof. Before that I had marched down the aisle with the sausage kings in tow demanding to see where the Chinese Bibles were kept.

"No vicar, not that I have come to terms with the yellow peril. It's actually about a lady."

"Ah, the fairer sex; much more complex than the yellow peril as you call it."

"It's been well over three years since I split from the wife vicar. Or rather, since she showed me the door and in all that time I have been like one of your Roman Catholic contempories minus the young boys of course." The vicar coughed at this but said nothing. I went on, "now I have finally met the most fantastic lady I could ever hope to meet. I love everything about her and she feels the same about me. She even thinks CROUCHING is cool."

"Who wouldn't?" Chipped in the vicar.

"Well yes," I went on, "anyway the thing is vicar is that she's married and she has young kids and she might be seriously ill and she's bordering on alcoholism and she's short and she..." The vicar held up a hand to stop me.

"Whoa Kirkland. Slow down. That's a lot of ands."

"And she doesn't measure her children's heads regularly," I mumbled under my breath.

"You say this lady is married?" The vicar suddenly had a serious vicar like expression.

I knew that would be the one he focused on. "She is, yes. But very unhappily so."

"But married all the same. You know the vows Kirkland. Marriage is a vow made before God. It is His witnessing of it that makes those vows sacred. You know I could never condone you interfering in another couples marriage."

"What if I was to tell you he beats her with a stick?"

"Does he?"

"I don't know. He may do."

"Come come Kirkland. You cannot cling to such absurdities. You must let these people; this family, sort their own problems out, God willing. Nothing good can ever come out of meddling in another man's marital affairs. Nothing but pain for all involved."

"But I love her vicar."

"Are you prepared to stand in front of a man, a wife, and their children and say that you are there to tear them all apart? Because that is what you will have to do and you won't have God on your side my son. Can you honestly say to me right now that you are strong enough to do that? Mentally strong enough?" He placed a large hand on my shoulder and added, "love can be a curse as well as a blessing."

"She loves me though vicar, it's not a one way thing."

"As I just said, love can be a curse."

I took a deep breath and looked up to the vast roof above me. The stone columns that reached up to it demonstrated the great craftsmanship of the stonemasons 700 years ago. I could only dream of having such a solid structure around me. "So what do I do? I'm not prepared to let her go."

"Are you prepared to wreck her family? Maybe ruin her children's upbringing?"

I sat in silence for a few moments then looked down at my feet. "No, I don't think I could deal with that," I answered honestly. "I don't think I'm ready for all that entails."

"Indeed, it is a huge decision to take on another man's family even for an emotionally strong person. I hate to say this but you know that you're not."

"Of course you're right vicar. I'm no way strong enough but I really couldn't face losing her either.

"So what you are saying is that you want to have your cake and eat it."

I laughed. "Yeah, I suppose I do."

"And you are worried this lady may one day soon, turn up on your doorstep with her bags and her children?"

"I cannot even be a father to my own son let alone someone else's."

"It seems like your head is telling you what your heart is refusing to hear."

"Believe me vicar, my head tells me all sorts of things."

"Now that I do believe, young man. It is a cross you have to bear. Mental illness is a terrible burden for many. Just remember that God will always watch over you but he cannot make your decisions for you. Only you can do that."

"Thanks vicar, you've been a great help." I went to stand up but he put a hand on my shoulder.

"Come; let us say a short prayer together."

I let him say his prayer and I even said 'Amen' at the end but I wasn't listening. I got up off the uncomfortable pew and thanked him all the same.

The old man smiled and said, "come and see me anytime Kirkland and think on about our conversation. Remember there are lives involved."

I thanked him again and went to leave but stopped at the last minute and turned to ask, "tell me vicar, is anal sex a mortal sin?"

CHAPTER TWELVE

THE GOOD FRIDAY MIDGET HUNT

CROUCHING Community Membership 4,869

That evening Big Andy dropped over my outfit that I had previously tried on with Craney, along with a couple of dubious looking Viagra pills and a large rope. He stayed for a beer and chatted to me and Gemma about the following day. I think he had a soft spot for Gemma and always came over a bit shy whenever he was in her presence. He didn't stay long as he had a couple of other outfits to deliver and as I waved him off he blew an air horn out of the transit's window. Gemma was laughing when I went back inside, busily inspecting my outfit and wearing my hat

"How dare you wear the sheriff's hat," I said in mock astonishment and grabbed it from her, much to her displeasure. We went back into the kitchen and over a couple of beers I told Gemma about my 'x' rated lunchtime activities whilst she sat through a children's matinee. She was upset that Uncle Percy hadn't been in attendance but was impressed by the 'bum love' as she called it and the shower sex. "Good girl," she had laughed. When I went on to describe my chat to the vicar she was less impressed; she had never been a fan of the church but when I told of my parting line she nearly spat a mouthful of beer over me.

"You never fucking did," she gasped.

"Of course I did Gem, what do you take me for?"

"You're destined for hell mate."

"I've already been Gem." I actually think I had.

A couple of hours later Gemma had gone to bed and once again I was left banging away at the keyboard like a man possessed, whipping up a fervour for the fast approaching midget hunt. I had arranged for all midget sightings to be relayed to a specially set up 'Midget Hunt' web page and asked people to post photos and videos as soon as possible. It appeared that hunting would be taking place all over the country with many cities taking up the challenge, including Liverpool, London and Bristol. However, it was my local hunt which I was now focusing my attention on, knowing that we had to lead the way. After a solid three hours of finger tapping I was finally satisfied that there was little more I could do before the big day, so I made my final pre hunt post:

There are only a handful of times in one's life when we are asked to stand up and face our most dangerous foes and greatest fears. Tomorrow is one of these times. None of us know how we will react when faced with a cornered large headed dwarf waving his short arms in anger or whether our nerve will hold when a crazed midget evades the lasso and makes a run for it. What we do know though is that fear will be our companion and God will be our guide. Together we can make this the most important Good Friday since the Romans nailed some poor bastard to a cross. LET'S GO MIDGET HUNTING!!!!

Kirkland Christie   Head of the CROUCHING Community

I awoke to the sight of the big shoe gleaming next to my bed and was immediately filled with a rush of excitement. My sleep had again been one of hallucinatory dreams and soaking wet sheets. Indeed, I was absolutely dripping in sweat as I pulled back the curtains.

To my delight the sky was cloudless. It was a gorgeous spring morning. I quickly showered and spent half an hour walking around the house in my boxers and the big shoe. Gemma was already rushing about packing bags and generally getting stressed about making sure she had everything together for her trip to Cornwall. From what I could see so far she may as well have just moved the whole house. The girls were over excited and winding their mother up and along with me stomping around in the big shoe she was at boiling point. "Will you all shut the fuck up?" She bellowed from the kitchen.

I took this as a good point to good back upstairs and get dressed into my midget hunting outfit. It consisted of a long black 'Wyatt Earp' sheriff's frock coat complete with a fancy black waistcoat. A black shirt and jeans and a great pair of black leather boots complete with spurs. Topping it all off was a fancy black Stetson, a shiny silver star and an old rusty pocket watch which Craney had found at a building site. I turned the hands to ten past ten. I also had a gun belt with a holster that had to be strapped onto my thigh just like a proper western gunfighter. The realistic gun was a water pistol. There would be a wide range of various water firing guns to keep meddling bystanders at bay. And most important of all was a long rope lasso for catching the midgets before they could run away. I put on my dark glasses and popped a big cigar in my mouth, this time a present from Big Andy and stood admiring myself in the mirror. "I am the law!" I shouted as I strutted around the bedroom, over the moon with my sheriff's outfit. On top of all this I hadn't even blown my bugle yet.

When the girls saw me they went crazy, shrieking in delight and pleading with Gemma to let them go midget hunting. The fact that I was still shouting "I am the law" didn't help. Eventually Gemma cracked and told me that I had 'five seconds to get the fuck out of her house before she attacked me.' I had seen Gemma lose it on a number of occasions and I wasn't about to push my luck on such an important day. I shouted to her to have a great holiday and made for the front door. I climbed the steps, taking time to look disapprovingly at the now barren front garden and sat down on the low wall with my legs stretched out across the pavement. The morning sun was pleasant on my face and I used the time to light my cigar. I puffed away contentedly even saying "good morning mam" to a woman across the road as she got into her car. She stopped to look at me and smiled a little nervously. I added, "it's a fine day for midget hunting wouldn't you say?" in my best Texan drawl. She quickly pulled open the car door and made a hasty getaway. I could see how difficult it was going to be to catch a midget when even people of normal height were so edgy around just me, let alone a dozen of us.

I decided to ring Craney to see if I could be picked up early. After a 'strange' conversation I think he said they would be about twenty minutes so I decided to take a slow walk in the direction they'd be coming. I had various strange looks from dog walkers and passing car drivers, as well as a group of kids kicking a football in the middle of the road. One of them shouted, "where's your fucking horse?" I stepped out to face them and soaked the mouthy lad with a couple of well aimed squirts from the pistol.

"I'm the sheriff in these here parts son and today I'm leading a posse of midget hunters."

"Fucking weirdo," the boy shouted at me, wiping his eyes, just as Big Andy's transit pulled up beside me. Craney jumped out of the passenger door, looking instantly menacing dressed in a full nun's habit and veil, a huge steel cross in his hand, false teeth and thick pebble glasses. The group of kids took one look at him and ran off in sheer panic. Big Andy threw him a pump action water gun out of the van window and I watched him chase after the fleeing kids which lasted about fifty yards before he realised he was completely wasting his time. He strolled back to the van and climbed in next to me.

"We're gonna have problems with him sheriff," said Big Andy leaning across me and trying to punch Craney in the side.

"I'm just doing the church's work," replied Craney, his hand worryingly disappearing up inside his habit. "Get back in your fucking cave."

Craney was referring to Big Andy's get up which was basically Fred Flinstone with a huge club which could have been made of papier mache or just as easily of oak. His large physique lent itself to the leopard skin wrap around 'outfit' and his only concession to modern day wear was a pair of size 13 steel toe capped work boots. He managed to argue with Craney all the way to the Josh and the pair of them didn't stop until we pulled up behind Sideways Stan's small red van, which had a St George's flag hanging over the back window with the words 'achtung midgets!' painted across it in thick black letters. Stan got out as he saw us and was dressed resplendently in a Superman get up but was quickly overshadowed when Dan jumped out of the passenger door wearing a huge papier mache head complete with crazy smiling expression.

"I'm Roger the midget," he shouted out from inside the huge head. Until that point we didn't even know it was Dan. Craney was over excited at the sight of this huge headed freak and the pair of them scuttled off to worry some shoppers. I could hear Craney shouting "nobody worry, I will catch the large headed freak," as Lenny and Carter arrived. Carter was leaning out of the taxi window blowing ear shattering noises from a rusty trombone and I could see the taxi driver shouting over his shoulder at him. Lenny, wearing some sort of 1970's floral dress and afro wig, his face blackened with boot polish left him too it and came over to me shaking his head.

"Morning mam," I said still in my Texan drawl. "Is that there some sort of Injun contraption?" I nodded towards the Ipad he was carrying.

"I need a fucking drink," replied Lenny. "Carter's been blowing that thing all the way up here. I thought the cabbie was going to hit him at one point."

Carter, still blowing the trombone marched over to us dressed in a full red British army uniform as in the Victorian days. He looked ready to make a last stand at Rourke's Drift.

"I thought we were after midgets not Zulus," laughed Big Andy as Carter finally ended his cacophony.

Carter was just about to reply when another cab arrived, this time carrying a full complement of four hunters. I watched in pride as a surgeon, a vicar, a Red Indian and another cowboy got out, all four carrying ropes made up into lassos. I gestured for everyone to go into the pub and then shouted to Craney and Dan to do the same. Craney had managed to lasso Dan and was shouting "I've caught the large head freak!" to amazed onlookers who had stopped their morning shopping trips to observe these strange shenanigans.

We went into the bar and were soon joined by a couple of clowns, Spiderman and a Germans SS storm trooper; much to Craney's jealousy. Lenny was busy pouring over the Ipad with me standing at his shoulder checking we were linked into the community website for 'midget sightings updates.' Almost an hour had passed and the hunters were beginning to get restless; although the consumption of beer was helping, before Lenny made the call: "Midget seen working at the Sainsbury's petrol station; Marsh Mills. From James T at Plymouth University."

I put the bugle to my mouth and let out a strangled blast. "Midget ho!" I shouted at the top of my lungs. Carter added, what sounded like a cat being run over on his trombone and with an air of nervous excitement we poured out of the pub to the vans.

"Man the wagons," shouted Craney who appeared like he was about to keel over from sheer excitement. He pulled open the back doors of the transit and showed off the somewhat chopped up sofa and chairs jammed in the back. I left him to it and climbed in the front with Lenny, as Big Andy started the engine. Sideways Stan did the same in his smaller van, shouting to Dan and his huge head to hurry up and get in the back. After what seemed like an eternity we finally headed off in search of our first midget. The Good Friday Midget Hunt had begun.

What should have been a five minute journey, ten at most, ended up taking almost half an hour as Craney decided to jump out of the back of the transit when we pulled up at the first set of traffic lights we came to. He ran through the queuing traffic to reach Stan's van which was a couple of cars behind us and wrenched upon the back door to get at Dan. Much to the amazement of the gawping onlookers Dan pushed past Craney and made a break for it shouting something about nobody ever catching the water melon head. With angry shouts and car horns ringing out Craney managed to stop three lanes of traffic by holding up his cross as Dan careered up the middle of the main road. Big Andy was cursing Craney out of his window, shouting that he was 'going to break his scrawny fucking neck' and eventually drove through the red lights in order to park the transit on the small grass verge that ran alongside the road. A minute or so later Sideways Stan did the same, the back doors of his van swinging wildly as he bounced up over the kerb.

"Right, I'm going to fucking kill him," snapped Big Andy as he opened his door and stomped in the direction of Craney and Dan who were now rolling around in a grapple of sorts in the central reservation. It was a ridiculous sight and cars were slowing down almost to a crawl to see what was going on. At least this allowed Big Andy to get across the road without any trouble and I heard Craney shouting, "I've secured the large headed beast" at him as he approached them. Ten seconds later Big Andy was marching back across the road with Craney over his shoulder who was screaming out, "Roger the midget is escaping," over and over. What the passing drivers must have thought as they saw a huge caveman carrying a nun over his shoulder, followed behind by some bloke wearing a huge papier mache head was any ones guess. I heard the Transit's door open followed by a loud thud and a scream from Craney and a minute later Big Andy was pulling off the verge and the hunt was back on.

The car park at the supermarket was packed; no doubt people stocking up for the long Easter weekend. Big Andy looked at me and raised his eyebrows. I pointed to the petrol station at the side of the huge supermarket, which was also busy; a long queue of cars waiting to get to the pumps. Big Andy eased the van into the queue, Stan following right behind us and I turned and banged on the dividing metal between the cab and the back of the van and shouted, "two minutes lads." I could hear the murmur of excited anticipation from within. However, it soon become apparent that it was going to take a lot longer than two minutes for us to reach the pumps, so mindful of Craney's complete lack of self restraint, I got out, along with Lenny, leaving instructions with Big Andy and headed to the petrol station shop in search of the reported midget.

Again I found dozens of heads turn in our direction as I stood outside the shop talking into Lenny's camera. In my best Texan drawl I said, "today is a historical day. I stand here as the sheriff responsible for rounding up midgets on the inaugural Good Friday Midget Hunt. Inside this here gas paying post I believe there to be a midget of unspecified head measurements and me and my posse are duty bound to protect society from its evil ways." With these words I entered the busy shop, Lenny following, still filming, and quickly looked around the place. I soon spotted the midget, the information had been right. She was behind the counter using a stool to reach up for a packet of cigarettes. A display of chocolate bars partially hid her body and it was impossible for me to make an accurate judgment on her height. At least one thing was clear; her head appeared to be the correct size in proportion with the rest of her body. I let out a sigh of relief then gave a robust "morning mam" to a woman who was staring openly at me.

The queue was six deep as I joined it, nodding to a couple of kids searching through the shelves of sweets. They looked up at me and giggled and I made an imitation gun with my fingers and pretended to shoot them, which they seemed to think was great. It was a good job Craney wasn't with me as he would have just blasted them straight in the face with his pump action gun. By the time I finally reached to counter I could see a few of the hunters wandering towards the shop and Dan with his huge head go running past with Craney chasing him. I ignored them and focused on the task in hand. I waited patiently as the midget did something with the till and tried to judge her exact height. She was sat on a tall stool which made it a little difficult for me. She didn't appear to be extremely short but she was definitely in my midget range. When she finally turned to me I touched the brim of my hat and in my best John Wayne impression said, "good day miss."

The midget looked up at me, offered a slightly toothy smile and replied, "Hello cowboy."

I refused to be taken in by her trickery of good natured banter and went on, "I'm the sheriff around these here parts and me and my deputies are rounding up midgets today."

Lenny was filming to the side of me and I could hear him snigger. I also caught the sight of Dan's huge head go racing past the shop again, in the corner of my eye. The midget had also seen this and for a moment stared open mouthed at the scene outside. Then she turned her attention back to me and said, "you must be that idiot who's always going on about midgets online. I've heard all about you."

"I don't know about that miss," I drawled. "Are you intending to come quietly or do we need to get the sacks?" As I said this, for once Craney's timing was perfect as he too ran past the shop waving a sack in the air and shouting some random nonsense. The midget was about to say something when there was a fracas involving Big Andy and a driver of a nice looking Mercedes who was pointing a finger and shouting something. From out of nowhere

Carter appeared and squirted water in the guys face. A chorus of 'midget fanciers' rang out as more of the hunters joined in drenching the Mercedes owner and then another poor chap who was nothing to do with it.

"I've pressed the panic button' said the midget to me. "It's linked directly to the police and the security people in the supermarket."

"I am the law!" I shouted at her pointing to my star, just as I saw Sideways Stan in his Superman outfit lasso the Mercedes driver, which led to a blast from Carter's trombone and a round of cheering from the rest of the hunters who were all in view now, bar Dan and Craney. Things quickly deteriorated as three security guards came running across to tackle the gunfighters and with a moment of inspiration I leaned across the counter, ignoring the protestations of the midget and grabbed the microphone that was linked to the speakers hooked up on the petrol station forecourt. I pushed down the red button beside it and said in a slow, calm drawl, "this is the sheriff speaking. Would all midget sympathisers and non hunters please vacate the forecourt for your own safety? There is a midget loose and we are here to catch it."

The midget was back on the phone and just as I was about to make a lunge for her a large pair of hands grabbed me and pulled me away from the counter. I still had the microphone in my hand and I just managed to shout, "help deputies!" Before it fell from my hands and two security guards firmly grabbed hold of me.

Within seconds Lenny had unleashed his water pistol into their faces and a vicar, Spiderman and Indiana Jones came to my rescue, bursting into the shop to the shock of the customers who so far had just been bemused by the whole affair, probably assuming we were a stag party or similar. After a brief burst of intense water jets and some wrestling I was pulled free and the five of us streamed back out onto the forecourt where big Andy was still arguing with various car owners. I grabbed the bugle from the inside of my frock coat and gave it a short strangled blast. "Retreat! To the wagons!"

Craig, who was dressed in an American grid iron outfit, had managed to block off two more security guards and Craney reappeared waving his cross around in front of him like a nun possessed, shouting, "the large headed one is dead, the large headed one is dead!" I didn't have time to ask him what he was on about but just grabbed him and pushed him towards the parked up vans. Eventually we were all back inside bar Dan who we picked up on the way out of the car park. He topped all else that went before when he was running across the car park waving at us and crashed straight into a shopping trolley. He was sent flying, his legs almost horizontal in the air due to the weight of the massive head. He was still on his hands and knees moaning; trying to lift his huge head as we reached him .Of course Craney jumped out of the van and pulled the head off. He then ran around the vans shrieking in delight and holding it aloft. "I have the large head!" he shouted over and over before Carter and Stan wrestled him into back of the transit minus the head. They threw it and Dan into the back of Stan's van and we finally headed off back to the pub empty handed but happy. We had barely had chance to order a pint when Lenny announced, "midget sighted on the Hoe, update to follow,"

"Okay boys," I said loudly, "make this a quick one. We may be off at any minute."

The laughter at our first attempt to capture a midget filled the bar and as other members of the CROUCHING community arrived, keen to get involved, Lenny made the announcement we'd all been waiting for and fearing: "Confirmed sighting on the Hoe. Large headed variety; wearing a yellow jacket and very short trousers."

A shiver went through me as I took in this news but I put the bugle to my lips all the same. I managed a fairly good hoot and shouted, "midget ho! Man the wagons."

It took about ten minutes to get everyone together which did little for my nerves. On top of having to face a large headed midget I also had to leave the sanctuary of Plympton. The Hoe, Plymouth's famous waterfront was about four miles away and thus quite a bit outside my comfort zone. But this was the midget hunt and I was the sheriff. I tried to focus on the task ahead rather than where it would be taking place. Lenny helped in this by giving me an update of all the latest news from hunters around the country. I was quietly amazed that other people had taken up the call with such zeal. The first one was from Liverpool, where apparently a large headed dwarf had been seen walking a dog that was bigger than him. Four hunters were on their way. There had also been sightings in Portsmouth, Bristol and

Swindon. A photo appeared of a midget in a Toys R Us store in London with a couple of teenagers waving plastic swords at it. I was just admiring this when my mobile buzzed. It was Carter saying that he needed more water for his water pistol. I directed big Andy to Elphinstone car park where I knew we could use the public toilets. It was just at the beginning of the long road that ran along the sea front and would be a good place to get a plan of action together.

Thirty minutes later we still hadn't reached the car park. It appeared the whole of Plymouth had decided to head to the Hoe for the bank holiday. The traffic was a nightmare and I could sense the unrest of the hunters who would probably be thinking how they could be enjoying a cold pint rather than be crawling along at a snail's pace in a cramped van. Eventually we reached Elphinstone car park and the hunters streamed out of the vans to both relieve themselves and refill their various guns. When everyone had both 'emptied' and 'refilled' we stood in a haphazard circle and I spoke with unusual seriousness, although I still did so with my Texan drawl. "Okay guys, we let the last one get away. This time we need a result. However, I don't need to remind you that the sightings we have all suggest that this one is of the large head variety. This is going to be a high risk adventure guys. Craney, no fucking it all up this time. Wait until you hear the bugle then go after it with the sack. Don't get second thoughts, just bag the bugger."

Craney saluted me, "aye aye Sheriff. You can count on nun Craney."

I shook my head and smiled. "Yeah right. Let's go then guys, happy hunting. Keep your eyes peeled and your ropes handy. We're looking for a short fella in yellow trousers and a fucking great head." With a blow from Carter's trombone and to the bemusement of the dozen or so fishermen lining the quayside we climbed back into the vans.

A few minutes later we were back in the crawling traffic, slowly making our way along the front sea wall of Plymouth Hoe. The pavements were heaving with people, long queues reached back from the cafe's and ice cream vans. I looked back and forth, my eyes straining for the sight of a midget. There was a bit of light relief when we stopped next to a group of Chinese people and let out loud shouts of "show us your sideways fannies" but other than this there was little to amuse us as we all became increasingly impatient.

"Midget captured in Leeds," exclaimed Lenny excitedly. "You won't believe the pictures."

I was getting agitated now. It wouldn't look good at all if midgets were caught around the country but not here. Plymouth was the stronghold of midget persecution after all. I needed a capture and quick.

"A bloke's been arrested in Liverpool for trying to bundle a midget into the back of his Ford Fiesta," Lenny shouted even though I was right next to him.

"Class," said big Andy, the first words I had heard him say since we left the pub, followed by a loud "cunt!" at someone on a bicycle trying to cut in front of him.

I was pondering on Sir Francis Drake who had famously played bowls here before sailing off to destroy the Spanish Armada over 400 years before. He had shown amazing patience, insisting on finishing his game first. It was just then, as we reached West Hoe, with its small but pretty park that I caught a glimpse of what may or may not have been our target. I pointed to big Andy who had a better view from his side but even he was struggling to see through the bustling throngs of people gathered around the large bouncy castle that was always busy on a day like this. After a minute or so I decided to get out for a better look and motioned to Lenny to do the same. I walked across the one way road and stopped at the picket fence and peered into the throng in front of me. The fact that there were about fifty kids running around didn't help, but then, at last, I saw him. "Midget Ho!" I shouted at the top of my lungs and let out a blast on the bugle. At least fifty heads turned in my direction but my eyes remained fixed on the large headed dwarf who was in the process of buying a drink from a small van parked close to the bouncy castle.

I heard the sound of Carter's trombone behind me and before I knew it Craney ran past me waving a sack above his head and shouting, "I'm here to catch the large headed one!" I gestured to the van and Craney shouted, "there he is!" and clambered over the fence rather than use the gate which was right in front of him. People had stopped what they were doing to stare open mouthed in disbelief and the unfolding scene. What they saw was a man dressed as a nun waving a large cross in one hand and a sack in the other, bounding through the shrubs to reach the midget, who had by now realised what was unfolding. The rest of the hunters were now all coming across the street and following me in through the gate, whooping with delight.

"Get the ropes," I shouted to Sideways Stan but before any of us did anything, Craney managed to get the sack caught amongst the rosebush thorns and ripped it completely open. "Craney, you're fucking hopeless," Lenny shouted at him as he filmed the whole shambles.

"It's all under control," Craney called back and then fell into the bush.

To make matters worse the large headed midget had realised he was the target of this crazy bunch and had made a dash for it. He managed to zig zag through the deck chairs which were full of parents watching their children on the bouncy castle and climbed up onto it presuming he would be safe amongst the bouncing kids. He hadn't counted on Craney though, who had now scrambled out of the thorns, less his veil.

As Craney was still trying to sort the ripped sack out I made my way to the front of the bouncy castle aware that there was a seriously large number of eyes watching me, wondering what on earth was happening. I touched my hat and said in a calm but authoritative voice, "keep calm ladies and gents. I'm the sheriff around these hear parts and me and my deputies are here to take in the large headed midget. Now you must understand that he's a seriously dangerous little bugger so if you'd kindly let us get on with our business we'll soon have the area secure."

"He doesn't make the height limit," one of the hunters shouted from behind me, followed by, "he's going to take a child hostage," from another. This led to a blast of water jets aimed in the general direction of the midget but actually just drenched three screaming kids.

I held up my hand and said "easy boys," as I heard the shocked shouts of angry mothers but when Craney suddenly made a lunge to climb onto the bouncy castle a dozen jets of water shot past me. Craney immediately slipped off the wet surface and fell onto the grass below, where he was soundly drenched.

"Hold your fire!" I shouted, trying to be heard above the angry voices of angry parents and shrieking children. A sodden Craney finally managed to stand up only for Sideways Stan to throw a perfect lasso over him to a load whooping. "Don't panic children I've secured the mad nun!" he shouted excitedly.

"Let me at the midget!" Craney shouted back as another round of water jets and a pull of the rope sent him crashing to the ground for the third time in five minutes.

The whole scene was one of chaos. There was now people streaming towards us from everywhere and I knew that we were rapidly running out of time to catch the midget. I was damned if I would let another slip the net and I pushed past the sprawled Craney, ignoring his pleas to lift him to his feet and walked to the closest point I could to address the midget who was now hiding amongst the children at the back of the bouncy castle.

"Son," I called. "You with the oversized head. You can't use these children as human shields. I'm the sheriff around these here parts and today I'm rounding up midgets. Are you going to come quietly?" I knew by the size of his head that he wouldn't give himself up but before I could shout for a rope I heard the booming voice of Carter above all the other commotion going on behind me.

"He's called for protection sheriff! The rival law enforcers are here!"

I turned to see a couple of women police officers were coming through the gate into the park. Over their shoulders I could see big Andy climb into the transit, which was causing all sorts of traffic problems, gesturing that he was going around to the other side of the park. I just caught the glimpse of Sideways Stan running across the road to his van when half a dozen women and a couple of blokes grabbed hold of me for the benefit of our rival law enforcement agents.

The two police women were both at least ten years younger than me and glared sternly as they made their way past the hunters to shouts of 'midget fanciers' as they headed towards me. There was a loud blast from Carter's trombone as they reached me, which didn't enhance their overall mood. The hands that had grabbed hold of me quickly let go at the arrival of the WPC's and I was quick to make the most of this opportunity. My real concern was that I now had my back to the midget, a no no in anyone's book. I held a hand up to greet them and said in my best authoritative American lawman sort of way, "I'm the sheriff around these here parts ladies. As much as I welcome your help I reckon it'd be safer for you to stand aside and let me and my deputies go about our duties."

"I'm sorry sir?" One of the police women said whilst the other was talking to a number of the parents.

"We caught this here varmint trying to jump on the kiddies' bouncy castle." I pointed to Craney who was still struggling with the rope around him but had managed to get to his feet. "My deputies have hogtied him for you ready to take him to the county jail." As I pointed to Craney three jets of water sprayed into his face leading to a loud "enough" from the other WPC. This was inevitably followed by a chorus of "midget fancier."

Whilst all this was going on the melon headed midget had decided to make a break for it, seeing the arrival of the police as the perfect opportunity to make his escape. It was Craney who shouted first. "He's making a run for it." Then added "Look at his little legs go!"

Carter let out a huge blast on the trombone and I did the same on my bugle, to the stunned faces of the WPCs who were now looking increasingly pissed off, to put it mildly. I watched helplessly as the midget belied his small stature to fairly bolt across the grass in the search of safety. Craney however had no such reservations and immediately loped off after him swaying from side to side, his arms pressed tight to his body where the lasso still held fast. A roar of encouragement went up from the hunters which grew louder as the two WPCs rushed after him. I was surprised how far he got and how much ground he made up on the fleeing midget. He made a valiant attempt at wriggling free of the coppers, who had grabbed hold of the trailing rope causing him to fall flat on his face. Whilst one of them was busy with a pair of handcuffs which seemed pointless considering the rope and only caused her more problems than she anticipated. The other copper was also holding onto Craney and trying to call for back up on her radio. Craney himself did his bit for the rest of us but causing one hell of a struggle and shouting at the top of his lungs, "I'm a helpless woman of the church"

I didn't need to think twice and was blowing the bugle as soon as the coppers had chased off after Craney. "To the wagons!" I shouted as loud as I could, this time the sense of urgency was real. With a chorus of 'whoops' and 'yee haws' the hunters charged off in search of the vans, the fortunate outcome of Big Andy's decision to park up well away from the park was that the coppers had no idea what vehicles we were travelling in. Sideways Stan guided Carter to them by mobile phone and when we rounded a corner to the street the two vans were parked in, we saw him in the middle of the road waving the 'achtung midgets' flag which he had wisely pulled down off the back doors. Thirty seconds later all of us bar the two drivers were crammed in the back of the vans and we made our way back to the Josh on separate routes. Considering we had lost another midget and were returning empty handed once more, the hunters were in great spirits. I myself was fuming that we had let another slip out of our hands.

It took just twenty minutes for us to get back to the Josh and the pub soon filled with the voices of excited midget hunters. The noise rose another octave when we crowded around Lenny's laptop and viewed the latest escapade. I had no doubt that the footage would prove to be a massive You Tube hit and that Craney would soon become a sensation. Lenny then went on to rattle through all the latest hunt information from around the country. The news of these faraway incidents continued to fill me with pride. I was particularly proud to hear that a large headed midget had been caught in Birmingham and had his head painted red. I inwardly cursed that I had not thought of doing this.

As the beers flowed the subject of Craney's arrest was the sole topic of conversation.

"They surely won't charge him," said Dan holding his huge head under his arm.

"I hope they do," I replied. "Think of the publicity we'll get."

"He'll no doubt be charged with large headed abuse," added Lenny, not looking up from the laptop. "There's been trouble in Bristol. It's not exactly clear to be honest, but it looks like there's a crowd gathered outside Top Shop shouting 'midgets out.'"

I smiled and nodded. "People are really taking up the call to arms. Small arms. It's turning out to be a red letter day. The days when midgets can just run wild are coming to end." I was about to go into some lengthy speech when Nikki walked into the pub and burst out laughing at the sight of the hunting party and our wonderful costumes. I gave her a kiss and bought her a pint of lager, then asked if she wanted to join the hunt.

"You must be joking. You're all end up with Craney if you're not careful."

I shook my head and said, "Craney is a martyr to the cause. He has given his liberty to allow the hunt to go on. And on it will go." I climbed up onto a stool just as I had a week before when announcing a CROUCH. This time it was to honour my crazy pal. "Gentlemen, I would like to say a toast to Craney for his selfless martyrdom on the Hoe in his pursuit of a midget. He gave up his liberty in order to allow the hunt to continue. Let's raise a glass to him and praise his commitment to the cause." I raised my bottle of Pils above my head and the hunters and many others in the pub did the same. "To Craney," I said loudly and was greeted by a loud chorus saying the same. It was a poignant moment and I could see in the expressions of the faces looking up at me, they knew what Craney had done for the midget hunt.

Lenny had no new sightings for us and I took the opportunity of the lull in proceedings to sit at the bar with Nikki and Carter. The conversation quickly turned to my relationship with Lucy.

"She'll be putty in your hands in the sheriff gear mate," laughed Carter.

"She's already putty in his hands," added Nikki.

This caused Carter to place his pint glass down on the bar. "Really?" He asked looking at me in what I hoped was admiration.

I nodded somewhat solemnly and answered, "Uncle Percy has been to visit." I knew Carter would get my drift.

"Excellent," he said. "And how was Uncle Percy?"

"He was thrilled in all aspects of his visit."

Before Carter could add anything Lenny shouted out, "midget apprehended in Sheffield. Some sort of library incident. Police on the scene at Bristol Top Shop." This piece of news was greeted with a loud chorus of 'midget fanciers' from the drinking hunters. Lenny waited for a modicum of order before continuing his rolling updates. "Berlin. Large headed dwarf of Turkish descent hooked on a fishing line." A loud cheer rang through the bar. I was thrilled to hear that our European cousins were taking the midget problem seriously. Lenny went on, "Burnley; four hunters chased a midget into WH Smith and have him cornered in the graphic novel section."

When Lenny had finally finished his running commentary I took the laptop from him and made the following post:

As you will no doubt be aware from our recent video uploads, one of our hunters has been arrested following his brave attempt to capture a midget who he had cornered on a bouncy castle. Unfortunately his attempt ended in a predictable farce and the rest of us had to do a runner but his efforts won't go in vain. At the very least he will be able to shout 'midget fanciers' at the old bill all night. I would like to personally thank all of your efforts so far today and urge all hunters to have one final push this afternoon. I hear the sound of little feet running...

Kirkland Christie   Head of the CROUCHING Community

Lenny was getting loads of grief about where the next midget was going to pop up and it was nearly another hour before he finally shouted out the news we had all been waiting for.

"Double midget sighting at Tesco Lee Mill!" He bellowed across the busy bar. "No confirmed head sizes. Last seen in the fruit and veg section."

Lee Mill was a small village less than a couple of miles from Plympton. It was practically on our doorstep. I blew the bugle as loud as I could and Carter did the same on his trombone. Big Andy added to the cacophony by blasting Craney's air horn, practically deafening Nikki who was stood beside him.

"To the wagons!" I shouted and downed the last of my Pils. I grabbed Nikki and dragged her out of the pub. Her remonstrations were lost as big Andy and Carter bundled her into the transit. Again shoppers stopped to stare at our motley crew, pointing at Dan and his huge head and at Billy and Stan holding aloft the 'achtung midgets' flag. Even without Craney we were definitely a modern day 'wild bunch.'

I heaved Nikki up into the front seats of the transit where she sat between me and Andy. She was shaking her head and moaning in disbelief that she had been roped into our latest escapade. I ignored her and gave another blow on the bugle and was just about to shout something out of the window when Lenny shouted from the back of the van. "I've got a picture. It doesn't look like they have large heads. They were in the pet food section a couple of minutes ago." It was great to think the general public were sending us photos of our quarry.

"Interesting," I said to myself which caused Nikki to look at me and shake her head.

It took less than fifteen minutes to reach the large Tesco superstore and I indicated to big Andy to park at the far end of the car park where there was plenty of space and was near the exit in case we needed to make a swift getaway. As soon as we stopped I jumped out and had a look around the car park. It was fairly busy and we would have to get a lot closer to the store before having any hope of spotting the midgets. I made the decision that it would seem probable that the midgets may well be parked in the disabled bays directly outside the store entrance and on this basis told the hunters to take up positions around the dozen or so cars parked there.

"What's the plan of action Sheriff?" Asked Dan just as big Andy whacked him over the head with his club.

"I reckon we just settle down and wait it out. A midget stake out so to speak." Then I had a thought. Turning to Nikki I said, "why don't you go in and see if they're at the check outs yet? At least we will have an idea how long we'll have to wait."

Nikki shook her head and said, "I can't believe I've been roped into this. I knew I shouldn't have come up the pub." However after a load of urging from the hunters she eventually was persuaded to go inside.

I watched her go through the sliding doors and once again felt my heart speed up. I glanced behind me to see the 'achtung midget' flag being held aloft again and noticed the eager expressions on faces of the hunters. We were like a pack of hyenas waiting for our prey. Shoppers gave us a wide birth; children pointed at us and tied up dogs barked at us. It didn't help that Ben, in his flowery dress and wide brimmed pink hat was spraying each dog in the face with his pump action water gun. As for a quick, quiet and decisive midget capture, it just wasn't going to happen.

After a few minutes Nikki came back out looking ever so slightly embarrassed and told me that there was no sign of the midgets anywhere near the checkouts, so it was decided that me and Lenny would go inside for a scout around. I had that awful feeling in my stomach that the midgets had evaded us. A few minutes later, to the bemusement of the bank holiday shoppers the sheriff and his side kick roamed around the aisles asking if anyone had seen a couple of small looking varmints. We had been at it for ten minutes before Lenny tapped me on the shoulder and gestured to me to look up the aisle opposite. There beside the Heinz baked beans were two midgets of the non large headed variety. The woman was ever so slightly taller than the man and they appeared to be husband and wife. What a bonus I thought as I walked towards them. The man was in the process of moving a stool to enable him to reach up to get something from the top shelf. I considered kicking it away from under him just for the hell of it but resisted the urge. I was the sheriff and needed to act accordingly. Behind me Lenny said "normal headage. That's a relief," and flicked open his camera. I held my position for a few moments trying to ascertain what would be the best approach to tackle them. I knew the best option now that they were here would be for me and Lenny to return outside and wait to ambush them with the rest of the hunters. However, I was the sheriff and I had a duty to protect the general public.

I walked slowly towards them, my heart rate almost through the roof and stopped about six feet away. Lenny had stopped further back down the aisle and was now videoing the unfolding scene. I was on my own. I stood directly in front of their weird little trolley that looked more suitable for a child to push around and waited for them to notice me. This took a bit longer than I thought as they appeared to be having an argument about what brand of beans to buy. It took all my will power not to intervene and say something clever. Finally the woman won the argument and the little man passed her whatever it was she was pointing at and she took it off him and turned to place the tin in the trolley.

"Afternoon mam," I said slowly and coolly. I must admit the accent was getting better and better. She looked up at me and frowned, not quite sure how to react. I went on, "I'm the sheriff in these here parts and today is the Good Friday Midget Hunt. Are you aware of this?" I could hear Lenny sniggering behind me but I remained absolutely resolute and professional. I stood motionless waiting to see what sort of reaction I would get and I didn't have to wait long.

"We know exactly what you are," said the woman in what I can only say was a very aggressive manner. "You ought to be locked up. You're a disgrace."

As she said this I found myself staring at her head. It did appear a little on the large size and perhaps this explained her aggressive attitude. "My posse are positioned outside with ropes and midget sacks. I'm offering you the chance to come quietly mam."

At this she raised a small arm and shouted, "you keep away from us! Terry, call the police."

"I am the law!" I barked at them and pointed to my silver star. My shout made Terry jump about an inch in the air.

By now we had attracted a fair amount of attention and two female shelf stackers had come over to see what was going on. The elder of the two, a grey haired woman pushing sixty asked if everything was alright. Before the midgets could answer I turned to face her and said, "I'm the sheriff in these here parts and I'm here to round up these midgets."

There was an audible gasp from the two shelf stackers and the woman midget snapped, "how dare you. What the hell is wrong with you?"

"Get the manager Sophie," The grey haired shelf stacker said to her colleague, who went rushing off past Lenny, who was still happily filming away. As she did, more people had stopped to see what was unfolding and I knew that it was getting close to the point where I would have to act. I decided perhaps a compromise may help so I said, "perhaps we could just take your husband mam. A show of goodwill so to speak."

"Somebody get him out of here," the female midget snapped and I became aware of more people taking an interest in the standoff.

"There's no talking to some people," I said to the grey haired shelf stacker who just stared back at me with a sort of shocked expression etched on her face. At the same time I noticed the male midget was talking urgently on his mobile phone. "Lenny, call for back up. I think these little buggers are going to make a run for it."

"Now that's quite enough of that," said the shelf stacker. "I suggest you leave immediately before you get into serious trouble."

"I've called the police," added the male midget snapping his phone shut.

"Yeah, piss off you sick prick." This from his ever so slightly large headed wife.

I was just about to calm her down with a blast of cold water when a large pair of hands were planted on my shoulders and I was pushed away from my prizes. "Time to leave mister," a voice said in my ear. I guessed it was security so I shouted at the top of my lungs, "midget fancier!" At the same time another two security guards appeared, followed by a suited man who I assumed was the manager. More hands grabbed me and as I approached the check outs there was no sign of Lenny or any of the hunters for that matter. The manager stepped alongside me and I turned and shouted in his face, "I'm the sheriff. You're stopping me doing my legal duty!"

I saw Dan's huge head appear as he charged through the sliding doors, followed by a vicar, a spaceman, a nurse and some sort of spiv cum gangster. Carter brought up the rear blowing noisily on his trombone.

"They've got the sheriff," I heard somebody shout as more of the hunters ran into the store; water pistols and pump actions to hand. Soon a torrent of water was raining down over the security guards.

"Release the sheriff!" I heard Carter boom out.

I turned to see who exactly had been manhandling me, getting a face full of water as I did so. It was a man of about fifty five, thickset and stocky along with a younger man who was in the midst of being absolutely drenched by the attention of at least half a dozen jets of water. The two of them were no match for the full posse. As soon as the grip on me was released I drew my pistol and squirted the manager straight in the face, hard enough that his glasses fell off. He had a look of total shock etched on his face, a shock which grew further when big Andy attempted to lasso him. All around me was chaos, with shoppers fleeing from the melee and shop workers unsure what to do. The midgets had disappeared completely. Lenny grabbed my arm and said quickly that he had heard that the police were on their way which caused me to curse loudly. I quickly considered my options, fuming that my quarry had once again slipped my clutches. Just then, like a blessing from above I heard a cry of, "midgets ho!" But in all the confusion I had no idea where the voice had come from. Big Andy looked across at me but all I could do was shrug. Then I saw Dan's huge head go haring towards the far exit. However, in his undoubted excitement to head of the midgets, he ran straight into one of those passport photo booths and ended up rolling around on the floor his head coming apart in two.

"To the exit!" I shouted at the top of my lungs and somehow managed to get a strangled noise from the bugle as I charged off in the direction of Dan who was still on his hands and knees. As we ran past him I could hear him moaning something about his 'beautiful big head.' We poured out onto the forecourt, shouts of 'yee haw' ringing out, along with raucous blasts from Carter's trombone. I nearly got knocked down by a bright red BMW as I raced across the road to try and gain a better view of the disabled parking area. I ignored the angry blast of the car's horn as I could see one of our quieter members of the hunt,

Perry, dressed reasonably conservatively as a fisherman or something, waving a sack over his head as he ran from the opposite direction. I immediately saw the two midgets about twenty feet away from him scurrying into their car. Perry didn't quite make it and I saw him throw the sack at the car in frustration as it pulled quickly out of the bay and shot away.

"Fuck it," I snapped. "The little buggers have got away."

Two minutes after the car had disappeared from sight the first of three police cars raced into the car park. The Good Friday Midget Hunt was over.

CHAPTER THIRTEEN

THE SHORT ARM OF THE LAW

CROUCHING Community Membership 4,927

"What can I do for you gentlemen?" I asked the three policemen stood in front of me. My Texan drawl if anything was even more pronounced. "I am the sheriff of these here parts and I am grateful for your assistance but you could say you have kind of missed the boat."

One of the coppers was on his radio, talking some kind of police nonsense that made them feel important. Over his shoulder I could see two of his colleagues talking to the manager who looked like a drowned rat. I lit up a cigar and went on to the copper who I had just addressed, "you see gentlemen, the varmint over there with your buddies," I pointed to the manager, "physically attacked me and my deputies were forced to cool his anger down so to speak."

"Okay, cut it out right now," the young copper said. "All of you." He motioned to Carter who was making random noises with his trombone. "Just keep quiet."

The policeman who had been on the radio turned to me and said, "we have had numerous reports of anti social behaviour across Plymouth today. I presume we've found the culprits."

"Officer, look what they have done to my head," moaned Dan showing the third of the coppers the two broken pieces of his lovingly made head. "It was that bloke over there," he pointed to the manager.

"He threw a tin of beans and sausages at me," added big Andy. "And it wasn't even a Heinz one."

"You see what my deputies have had to deal with officer?" I added for good measure.

"Right, I won't tell you again. Keep it shut." Politeness was in short supply from our rival law enforcement agency.

A squirt of water passed over my shoulder and hit the copper on the side of his neck. Behind me I could hear a fit of giggling the like you would expect from a group of young school children. Someone also said "midget fancier," in a manner that could only have come from him trying to keep his mouth closed.

"Shut it!" The copper shouted obviously losing his patience. "Who squirted the water then?" He knew he wasn't about to get a reply. Then added after a few seconds and I may say somewhat smugly, "don't worry, you'll have plenty of time down the nick to tell me." I was proud of my hunters when this threat was simply met with more calls of 'midget fancier.'

I watched the manager and the other coppers disappear into the store, no doubt to speak to eye witnesses and view CCTV and the like. "Perhaps it would be wise to let my deputies on their way officers," I said. "I am more than happy to discuss a way of joining forces so to speak."

"None of you are going anywhere," replied the young copper. "You stay put until back up arrives, then we'll decide who's going where."

"So what you're saying is that you have no way of dealing with all of us at the moment?" I took my bugle from the inside pocket of my frock coat. "I could blow a retreat signal."

The copper took a couple of steps forward. "You blow that and you're nicked."

"Are you going to arrest me for blowing a bugle?" Obviously I blew it anyway, knowing it was the last chance for some of the hunters to evade the clutches of our competitors. I managed to shout, "to the wagons," before two coppers jumped on me. As I made the most of making it as difficult as possible for the two young constables to keep hold of me, I heard various shouts of 'midget fanciers' as I was wrestled to the ground, happy in the knowledge that, like Craney, I was sacrificing myself for the good of the hunters. Saying that, as a pair of hand cuffs were roughly applied, I got a face full of water as no doubt, some of my deputies were unhappy at my rough man handling.

"They've got the sheriff!" I heard Carter shout from somewhere, as more water was sprayed in the direction of my capturers.

"Save yourselves boys," I managed to shout. "Go after the midgets!" A large knee in the middle of my back put an end to my urgings. I heard myself grunt as I was slammed back down onto the tarmac. I continued to do my best to struggle but I was no match for my fully paid rivals. Eventually they pulled me to my feet and breathing heavily I said, "I'm too tall to be arrested." The remark was ignored as all attention was now focused on rounding up as many of the hunters as possible. I saw Carter being grabbed from behind, his trombone clattering to the ground and also saw Dan trying to carry his head and flee at the same time, only to be apprehended by two coppers running back out of the store. In the distance, somewhere behind me, I could hear the ominous noise of sirens heralding the arrival of reinforcements. I was pulled roughly towards a police car and shoved into the back and told to "shut the fuck up" in response to my ranting "I'm the sheriff" over and over again. All I did was shout "midget fanciers" instead. My repertoire wasn't very inventive but it did piss off the young copper stood at the car door beside me no end. I was expecting to be moved to the van for my trip to the cop shop but I was actually taken in the comfort of the car. I presumed this was due to my stature as a sheriff of the law.

Thirty minutes later I had been booked in and was settling into a fine example of luxury modern living in a cell at Charles Cross police station in Plymouth city centre. I had not been able to ascertain if Craney was here somewhere and despite my shouting at the cell door I had received no response. He was either asleep or at one of the city's other fine establishments. It was the best part of an hour before I heard big Andy shout, "Sheriff! Carter's been buggered in the toilets. And he enjoyed it! They played on his other trombone!" This was followed by some swearing, the sound of a struggle and the slam of a cell door. I could hear big Andy cursing something or another faintly in the distance. Over the next hour I heard various shouts of "Craney" and "midget fanciers" as more of the hunters arrived for the night. From what we could gather there was six of us in the cells. Along with me, Andy, Dan and Carter there was Questy and the rather unfortunate Tim. The banter went on for another hour before things started to quieten down, alcohol and nervous energy finally getting the better of the hunters. I went about my own business happily, practicing a number of 150 degree, left leg extension CROUCHES, in the middle of my cell.

It wasn't until I had been handed my evening meal; a sealed packet of ham sandwiches and a bag a plain crisps, by a burly looking female officer, that it dawned on me that I was meant to be spending the night with Lucy. I vented my frustration by administering a full rendition of animal noises, much to the delight of the other hunters and another loud chorus of "midget fancier" shouts. If I managed to get any sleep whatsoever I don't recall it. Most of the night was passed with me pacing the cell frantically, broken only with bouts of intermittent CROUCHES and calls of 'I'm the sheriff!' Nobody appeared to be listening. Except Carter that is, who spent most of the night shouting 'welease woderick' in his best Monty Python impression.

The thought of missing Lucy filled me with real concern. She would be heading off overseas in twenty four hours and the police had basically robbed me of my last night of fun with her. It was no doubt all part of the midget conspiracy that I had been fighting against right from the start. I wondered if the Chief Superintendent was of less than average height. I was in *this* unforgiving mood when my cell door was opened and I was handed a tray with a packet of cereal and some UHT milk for breakfast. I had barely finished it before the door was opened again and I was lead out to the custody desk. It was a different sergeant than previously but he still appeared to hate me with every fibre in his body. I was bailed to return in three weeks time and after signing some paperwork was handed back my wallet, keys, watch, phone and belt. For once I kept my mouth shut, too worried about Lucy still to think about much else. All I managed was a few nods and a murmured 'yes' about understanding the bail process before turning and leaving the police station. As I pushed through the doors I glanced at my watch. It was ten past ten.

I should have guessed I would have company once outside and sure enough I was greeted by all the rest of the now released hunters, bar Carter who appeared behind me shortly after I stepped out into the sunshine. What I wasn't expecting was a large crowd of students cheering loudly or the number of journalists jostling for a quote or a photo. I recognised a number of the students from recent CROUCHES and as the police station was slap bang in the middle of 'student land' I could understand their presence, but the press? I gave a thumbs up sign to the students and was about to speak to big Andy when four cameras were thrust in my face and an attractive woman about ten years younger than me clasped hold of my arm in an iron grip that defied her slight stature. She told me she was from the local TV news and wanted an interview. At the same time two men appeared with microphones almost pushing them into my face.

"Mr Christie, can you explain your actions yesterday that led to you being arrested?"

I placed my Stetson, which I had been carrying; back on my head and raised a hand up in a gesture that I hoped would imply all was fine. I turned to look directly into the largest of the cameras which I guessed was the TV one and said in my best Texan drawl, "well miss, me and my deputies were stopped by this here rival law firm," I gestured to the building behind me, "from carrying out our midget hunting duties."

"And these duties involved the kidnapping of midgets?" The reporter said 'midgets' as if she was swearing in the Vatican.

"Yesterday was the inaugural Good Friday Midget Hunt. The clue is in the title miss. We were hunting midgets not kidnapping them. Around the country and in many other parts of the world the CROUCHING community came together to try and do something about the terrible midget problem that is spreading across our towns and cities. Brave men and woman, dressed in a wide range of fancy dress costumes, went out to seek the large headed ones in particular, with a zeal that can only be commended." There was a large cheer from the students and a strangled noise from Carter's trombone which he had miraculously recovered.

"Mr Christie, how can you possibly justify such an act?"

"Well what exactly would you expect us to do on a midget hunt miss?"

"Are you aware that over twenty people across the country have been arrested for similar offences yesterday?"

I smiled broadly. "They have given up their liberty for your safety miss. The streets are a safer place to walk today. I will add though that many of these midgets must have friends in extremely low places."

"Surely you are not condoning what can be said at *best* is drunken anti social behaviour." I could tell the reporter was getting slightly annoyed at my stance but wanted to keep me talking.

"Tell me this miss. Are you some sort of midget fancier?" I said this in the knowledge that the calls of 'midget fancier' would no doubt ring out from the recently released hunters. They didn't let me down and better than that the students took up the call as well. For a couple of minutes it was impossible for the reporter to ask any other questions and before she could do so I shouted at the top of my lungs, "as long as I am the sheriff in these here parts I will do my utmost to keep the public safe from these marauding little buggers. I will now CROUCH for a short period." I immediately slipped down into a sublime 120 degree double knee bend, right foot turned ever so slightly inwards CROUCH and as expected everyone present bar the press and an uneasy looking constable who had appeared from the station entrance, followed suit. More questions were shouted by the assorted members of the press and more photos were taken but I ignored them all. When I stood back upright I shouted, "thank you all for your support and for attending today's CROUCH outside Charles Cross Police Station." I turned back to the woman reporter and smiled, touching my hat as I did so before looking directly into the camera. "For all you parents out there who are no doubt worried about your youngsters potential for large headed growth, just remember to measure your children's heads at least once a week and always check under your beds before turning off the lights." With this final offer of advice I pushed my way past the press and went over to the students to shake a few hands and thank them for their support. The press had their story and I had my community. All was good in the world. Then I remembered Lucy again...

It was ten past ten when Nikki pulled up outside Gemma's. I kissed her on the cheek and made my way wearily down the steps and into the house. Nikki had not really known what to make of yesterday's events. She had said that the internet was buzzing about the hunt and Lucy had 'pissed herself' when she had found out about my arrest. Gemma was less impressed and had wanted to end her long weekend break and drive straight home but thankfully Nikki had persuaded her not to. As I waved Nikki off I let out a sigh of relief at being home and more importantly that Lucy was not upset. She had left a number of messages on my phone telling me I was a twat and that she would find a way of seeing me before she went away, even if she had to come to the police station.

I resisted the urge to immediately sit down at the PC and instead went upstairs, stripped off and stood under the shower and didn't move for a long time. As I dried myself I caught my reflection in the mirror and saw how tired I looked. I considered crashing on the bed but instead, dressed, went downstairs and filled the kettle. I was in need of a few strong mugs of coffee. As I waited for it to boil I sent a text to Lucy telling her I was home and very randy. In actual fact I was anything but randy, however, it seemed the right thing to say. She replied within a few seconds saying that she would call me as soon as she got chance. I followed this by ringing Gemma and said a silent prayer of thanks as the answer phone kicked in. I left a slightly garbled message saying I was all safe and sound and that I had a couple of large headed midgets in her garage.

I went back upstairs to get the big shoe and spent twenty minutes walking lopsided back and forth across the front room carpet before finally succumbing to the pull of the computer. Nikki had not been exaggerating; the social media sites were abuzz with midget hunting stories and speculation. I spent an hour watching video footage of our exploits and then another hour watching the exploits from other hunts. The viewing was hilarious.

Craney was already becoming an internet sensation and no doubt would soon be the darling of 'You Tube.' I sent him a long message summing up what had gone down after his arrest and asked him to ring me when he got chance. Lenny had done a fantastic job of filming the day's events and to his credit there were already hundreds of comments under each of his recently uploaded clips. It would take all day for me to read through them all.

One thing that did make me laugh was the fact that we had made both the BBC and ITV local news. The reports were not very flattering but they did include a clip from Lenny's coverage of Craney's arrest, with me shouting 'I am the law' in the background. My parents would be thrilled. I grimaced at the thought of that conversation. Eventually I gave up trying to read anymore comments; it would have to wait for a long sleepless night and instead made a comment myself.

I would like to thank all of you who took part in yesterday's inaugural Good Friday Midget Hunt. The day was a tremendous success although my own local hunt was rudely interrupted by the short arm of the law, leading to my arrest along with a number of my hunting colleagues. I am in no doubt that that there will be midget fanciers up and down the country who will frown upon our fine efforts so I have a message for them: How would you feel if you woke up one day to find your middle class avenues over run by short people with huge heads and tiny arms? You will ask where is the sheriff when we need him most?

There will be a special Easter Sunday CROUCH tomorrow outside St Mary's Church in Plympton at ten past ten.

Kirkland Christie   Head of the CROUCHING Community

I was in the middle of making another cup of coffee when Lucy called.

"Hello yes?" I answered as per normal.

"Hey sheriff," Lucy replied in a sexy voice. "Did they bugger you all night in your cell?"

"If there's to be any buggering to be done it is to be done on you woman."

"Promises promises," Lucy answered immediately bringing a stirring to my groin.

"Well mam," I said reverting to the Texan drawl, "I have an empty house and nothing on but a Stetson and my holster. If you get here sharpish I may even slip on my cowboy boots."

"I'm trying to get everything done so I can get away for an hour or two. Try not to do anything stupid for a few hours and you might get to ride me instead of your horse cowboy."

"I know I mentioned the boots but in all honesty I think I may keep the big shoe on."

I could hear an audible sigh come down the line. "You know how to push all the right buttons. I wondered how long it would be before you mentioned the bloody shoe."

"Look, just hurry up and get here."

"Okay okay. I'll ring you as soon as I have done all my chores."

"Alright fat head. I intend to give you a real hard seeing to. You know, to keep you going so to speak."

"In that case I better pull my finger out lover boy. See you shortly." She added a naughty chuckle and hung up.

I grabbed a couple of pieces of Asda's own brand wafer thin ham and made the delayed coffee before sitting back in front of the computer. I wish I hadn't. There were a number of comments that were particularly disappointing. Words such as "disgusting," "scum," "bullies," "thugs," and worse were being aimed at us and in particular, me, from all angles. I couldn't understand what was wrong with some people. Fortunately there were many more comments that were positive and a large number that were positively ecstatic. If nothing else at least the midget problem was now firmly at the forefront of many people's minds. I had the real impression that with a good wind we may one day get the midget cull that was so obviously needed across the country. For the moment though, I had done my bit and could relax in the knowledge that our posse had not let anyone down. We had paid with our liberty and there was little more that we could have done.

I noticed that there was an awful lot of abuse appearing from midgets themselves. Some of it was foul and I mean absolutely foul. I was threatened with a whole host of violent ends to my life and torturous attacks. I assumed these to mean knee capping or similar. If only I had been able to get in touch with these midgets the day before it would have saved a hell of a lot of time hanging around for reported sightings. I was about to reply to a particularly nasty comment about my manhood when Lucy called to say she was on her way. I quickly put the threats to my cock and balls to the back of my mind and ran upstairs to brush my teeth and spray on a bit of aftershave. I was just placing the big shoe carefully onto my bedside chest of drawers when the door bell rang.

"Impressive," Lucy said as I pulled her hand against my erection before she had even made it into the hallway. The bulge in my jeans was indeed impressive; by my recent standards anyway. Lucy herself looked stunning as always. She was wearing skin tight black jeans with knee high black boots over the top. A tight black sweater clung sensuously around her breasts and was cut short to show off her belly button piercing. She let go of the 'bulge' and put her arms around me, reaching up to kiss me passionately. If anything the bulge got even larger.

"Get up those fucking stairs now," I ordered, breaking free of the embrace and manhandling her towards the staircase. She took no further encouragement and pulled me by the hand swiftly up to my bedroom. We were barely through the door before she was undoing the buttons to my jeans and sliding to her knees to take me in her mouth. She stared up at me as she teased the end of my cock with her tongue, her sparkling blue eyes searching out mine for a connection. She slapped my hand to get my attention as I had been staring at the big shoe trying to decide whether to give it to Zak as part of his birthday present. The slap reverted my attention and I placed both my hands on Lucy's head and began to pull at her hair. She murmured some sort of gargled encouragement and went at my cock with such vigour that it wasn't long before I had to pull her up and heave her onto the bed for fear of getting 'carried away' too quickly.

I told her to get naked and a minute later we were lying facing each, Lucy's hand stuck like glue to my stiff cock as we kissed longingly and hungrily. I winced as the nails of her free hand dug deeply into my back but carried on like a trooper as she told me in very basic English to 'suck my fucking tits you fuck.' Five minutes later she was riding me like I was the odds on favourite of the Derby and was spurting so much filth from her mouth I did at one point consider covering my ears. Twice she called me 'a dirty fucking shit eater' which was a new one on me. Regardless of all the abuse, or maybe because of it, I gave her a really good seeing to and we both came within seconds of each other. The special moment was sealed as she screamed "shoot your fucking spunk up my wet cunt you dirty fucking whore fucker!"

We lay embracing each other, Lucy's hair falling across my face as we caught our breaths, neither of us saying a word. We remained like this for fifteen minutes, both of us lost to our thoughts. Lucy no doubt thinking about her rapidly approaching holiday, me wondering if Craney would turn up for the Easter Sunday CROUCH still wearing his nuns get up? To my surprise and pleasure the old boy suddenly began to stir again as if by magic. I hoped it wasn't the thought of Craney that had aroused me but whatever the reason I was grateful. Lucy was over the moon. I threw her off me and took her aggressively from behind, letting out all my pent up fury at not catching a midget the day before. Predictably I had to shove Lucy's face into the pillow to shut her up but even that wasn't enough to stop her upsetting half the neighbourhood as she enjoyed her second and third orgasms of the day. By the time I reached my climax we were both dripping in sweat and puffing like we had just finished the London marathon.

Twenty minutes later we were sufficiently recovered to manage a cuddle and Lucy told me that I had undoubtedly just given her the best seeing to she had had in years. Indeed she had a look of someone intensely satiated. It did wonders for my self esteem. Yet we both knew that the subject of her holiday would have to be approached before much longer and it was me who eventually broached the subject.

"I'm going to miss you like hell fat head." Tears immediately welled up in her eyes and I tenderly kissed her on the forehead. "I don't know what I'm going to do without you here to amuse me."

"Wank?" She smiled through the tears.

"You know what I mean," I said, rubbing my hands gently up and down her back. "It's less than a week but I can't..." I didn't end the sentence; I didn't know what to say.

"I could have killed you last night when you got locked up. I was so upset when I couldn't see you." Lucy wiped away her tears. "Fuck knows how I'm going to cope being so far away from you." Now tears came again and this time she cried properly. There was little I could do other than hold on to her and wait. Eventually I said, "don't go worrying fat head; there's quite a few 21 year old students that are desperate to service their hero."

"Twat." Lucy said then carried on crying. She cried for another ten minutes which is quite a lot of crying in my book, before eventually pulling herself together and allowing us to have a proper conversation.

"The midget hunt made the news you know," I said proudly.

"I know. I saw you. You are famous at last."

"I told you it would happen. The CROUCHING community is a force to be reckoned with at last."

"I thought you looked very dashing in your sheriff's outfit. Who was the nun?"

I laughed, "Craney. Obviously. I haven't heard a thing from him since he got nicked."

"You lot really are all crazy. I couldn't believe it when Nikki rang me."

"You couldn't believe it?" I replied raising my eyebrows.

"Okay. Well yeah I could believe it. I was so stressed at the thought of not seeing you though. I could have killed you."

"You nearly just did."

She laughed loudly, all signs of the tears finally gone. "Imagine that? I would have been a pin up girl for the midgets."

I grunted, then shuddered at the thought of hundreds of midgets ogling Lucy. "I'm going to concentrate on CROUCHING whilst you're away. I need to reach back out to the core of the community. I don't want to alienate anyone. Fuck the midgets,' I've done my bit where they're concerned."

"I'm glad to know you'll be keeping yourself busy while I'm away."

"I'll have to be. It's going to be the longest week ever otherwise."

"Just promise me you won't end up behind bloody bars again."

I grinned and replied, "I'll try not to." Then added after a few seconds, "I really think I can do something special with the CROUCHING community fat head."

"I'm sure you can Kirk."

"No, I mean *really* grow it beyond all recognition. Make people sit up and take notice. Look how easy it's been with the midget hunt. I'm all over the press and on the box, let alone the hits on You Tube and Twitter." I clapped my hands together excitedly and said loudly, "28 people were arrested yesterday for midget related offences. That's incredible. All over the country and other countries for that matter, people went out and hunted midgets for the only reason that *I* said so." I stressed the 'I' as grew more impassioned by the second. "People had a great day out yesterday. Middle aged men put on fancy dress and went out in convoys to hunt midgets. The world is waking up fat head. And I am the pied piper calling the tunes."

Lucy stared at me with a concerned expression. "It's madness."

"Absolutely," I agreed, clapping my hands again. "My madness is now being adopted by thousands of others. It's contagious. People are using me to act out their madness."

"You're definitely *something* Kirk," laughed Lucy as I reached past her to pick up the big shoe.

"Doesn't it make you warm inside fat head?" I held the big shoe above us. "Knowing you are so close to a big shoe?"

"You and that fucking shoe. You really are obsessed."

"I'll let you smell the inside if you want. A kind of leaving present." I offered Lucy the shoe as if I was presenting her with a fine wine to taste.

"Fuck off!" She shouted and hid under the quilt. The next thing I knew she was playing around with my genitals so I put the big shoe carefully back on the chest of drawers and settled back down, closing my eyes in anticipation. I say closing my eyes but I did keep one half open. Too look at the big shoe obviously.

CHAPTER FOURTEEN

FAMOUS, INFAMOUS OR JUST PLAIN MISERABLE?

CROUCHING Community Membership 6,411

How long have you got?" I asked Lucy as we stood in the kitchen.

"I can't stay too much longer," she replied taking a drag on her cigarette. "Fuck, I hate this."

"Just don't go," I said trying unsuccessfully not to sound like I was begging. "Stay here with me and I will do all sorts of horrible things to you. I've got Viagra now you know."

"Oh Kirk, if only. Please don't make this any harder than it already is."

I poured us both a glass of wine at the same time noticing how sad Lucy looked. I knew this was hard for her but wasn't about to let her off the hook that easily. I took a sip of the atrocious wine, winced and through slightly gritted teeth said thoughtfully, "I promise not to sleep with anyone else whilst you are away."

Lucy looked at me with a pained expression.

"I won't, I promise," I reiterated.

"You are waiting for me to say the same?"

I shrugged. "Not at all, I was just letting you know that's all."

Lucy frowned deeply. "Kirk, don't start playing games. You know I don't do games."

"Okay, I apologise. I will in fact sleep with someone whilst you're away."

"Twat!" Lucy shouted and punched me on the arm.

"But what about the Viagra? It might go out of date."

"I tell you what. You keep the Viagra for when I get back and I will dress up in my sexiest undies and highest heels and you can do whatever you like to me." She winked mischievously.

"Will you wear the big shoe?"

"Twat twat fucking twat!"

I took hold of her hands and looked at her, peering over the tops of my shades. "Sweetheart I am going to miss you. Promise me you won't come back a different person."

"Different person?"

"Towards me."

She leant forward and kissed me tenderly. "I promise. You have nothing to worry about baby. I'm crazy about you. 100% crazy."

Twenty minutes later I watched her car pull away into the late afternoon sunshine. I suddenly felt lower than I had in ages. I was going to miss her one hell of a lot. Lucy had tried not to shed any more tears as she said good bye but I could see the wetness in her eyes. As she had stood in the porch I had held my hand out to her and when she clasped it I shook it and said, "well bon voyage and all that." She had called me a twat and rushed to the safety of her car. I could see that she was in floods of tears as she sped off. I just stood silently, dimly aware that I was in love and that my girl was about to sail off to France for a romantic break with her husband. Eventually I closed the front door and returned to the kitchen to spend the next few hours laying face down on the floor. It was only the incessant ringing of my mobile phone that finally brought me out of my deep sulk.

"Hello yes?" I answered wearily.

"Ah you are free man again then," Gemma's voice laughed into my ear.

"A great injustice has been thrust upon me Gem."

"For fuck's sake Kirk, I'd been gone less than five hours before Nikki calls and tells me you've been nicked."

"It's some sort of midget conspiracy. It wouldn't surprise me if the Chief Superintendent has a kid with a head the size of a beach ball." I gave Gemma a brief run down of the previous day's events. She was in hysterics. She didn't stop laughing until I got onto the subject of Lucy.

"She'll be back before you know it mate."

"I hope so Gem. It's going to be a tough week."

"Right, I am going to ring Nikki to come over and see you. I know you're on the bloody kitchen floor again." Gemma always knew.

She was good to her word and an hour or so later Nikki turned up. I was indeed still on the kitchen floor but had managed to go upstairs and grab the big shoe which was now placed beside me on the lino. I was staring at it when I heard a loud, "helloooo" signalling Nikki's arrival.

"How long have you been lying there Mr Christie?" Nikki said laughing and filling the kettle.

"Ever since Lucy ran off with her husband," I replied morosely.

"You've seen her then?"

"Yeah, she came over earlier, abused me three times and fucked off to France."

"Three times!" Nikki exclaimed as she fumbled about in the dishwasher looking for clean mugs. "That's about five years worth for you isn't it? I bet she couldn't believe her luck?"

"It was a very romantic session of love making," I grunted.

Nikki almost dropped the mugs. "What you mean is you slapped her arse and spunked over her tits."

"Yeah something like that."

I finally got off up the floor and took the mug of coffee Nikki offered me. We ordered a take away (obviously not Chinese although that was Nikki's preferred choice) and went and sat in the lounge. Nikki got straight onto the subject of my recent television appearance.

"You're famous."

"Infamous more like."

"It's a good job your son's away. Have you heard anything from your mum and dad?"

I grimaced, "not yet but it won't be long." I didn't want to begin to think about my mother's opinion on my new found fame. I quickly changed the subject. "Was the report fair do you reckon?"

"What do you mean by fair?"

"Did the reporter agree that midgets need hunting?"

"Uh, no Kirk."

I shook my head. "Liberal fucking press."

"Put the computer on, you can watch it yourself."

I agreed. "Okay, you do it. I need to reply to some of these texts. I've got loads of them." This was indeed true. Thirty six in all and everyone one appeared to be congratulating me on my recent exploits.

"Here it is," Nikki pointed excitedly at the screen.

I reluctantly put down my phone and turned my attention to the computer screen. The report started with the local BBC newsreader saying that a number of arrests were made today in relation to a so called midget hunt, blah blah blah. It was the usual BBC nonsense, all fact and none of the fancy embellishments needed to fabricate such a great story. Imagine what the much missed 'News of the World' would have done with such a scoop. The clip moved from the studio to outside the Charles Cross police station and all of a sudden there I was in full sheriff mode. Nikki was already roaring with laughter and I had to shush her so that I could hear what the reporter was saying. To their credit the BBC broadcast unedited my speech about making the streets of Plymouth safer and the fact that the reason midgets were so dangerous was due to their short arms and large heads. All in all it was an excellent piece of publicity and I was cheered no end. The report finished with the newsreader saying that three men in Manchester had been arrested for allegedly hanging a midget off a bridge by his legs.

"It's a shame we didn't make the national news," I muttered to Nikki. "You'd think the BBC would get their priorities right wouldn't you? Bombings in the Middle East are so fucking predictable. For Christ's sake, there is evil lurking on our very own streets."

Nikki finally stopped laughing and asked, "so you haven't finished with the midgets then?"

"Not in the slightest. Although I am going to focus on CROUCHING again for the moment. There's a huge one taking place in New York tomorrow."

"Conquering the world eh?"

"Damn right Nikki. Conquering the world." I raised my mug as you would toast with a wine glass, at the prospect of witnessing people CROUCHING all over the world except China.

Our take away arrived and our conversation turned back to Lucy. By the time she left, Nikki had persuaded me not to worry about her and that she would be home before I knew it. I felt a good deal more positive and made myself comfortable in front of the computer pouring over the reams of comments relating to the recent news broadcast. Nikki was right – it was indeed big news. There was a real opportunity to create a bit of momentum so I put Lucy firmly to the back of my mind and concentrated at the task in hand. I made the following post:

As the head of the CROUCHING Community it is often said that I spend too much time lying face down on the kitchen floor and not enough time exploring new CROUCHING venues. I am therefore pleased to announce a new CROUCHING venue for each day of the next week. This will begin with a high noon CROUCH outside Comet Superstore on Marsh Mills, Plympton, tomorrow. This is in addition to the already announced Easter Sunday CROUCH outside St Mary's Church at ten past ten. So make sure you keep up to date with the website for each new venue. Also and this is vitally important – after the huge success of yesterday's inaugural midget hunt, keep your eyes pointed downwards in case of any potential midget backlash. Keep measuring your children's heads and always check under your bed before switching off the lights.

And it goes without saying, strictly no Chinese at any of the forthcoming CROUCHES.

Kirkland Christie   Head of the CROUCHING Community

I counted over forty messages of abuse aimed at me relating to the midget hunt. Quite a number of them were very threatening. A shiver went down my spine as I wondered whether any of the threats were from large headed dwarfs. "Evil little fuckers," I said to myself as I re-read a particularly nasty one. Thankfully there was three times the amount from well wishers, many of whom were overseas. Russians, in particular, seemed to have taken to the midget problem very seriously. A photo from a chap called, somewhat wonderfully Big Ivan showed a large man with a massive gingery beard, running across a football pitch with an elderly midget under his arm. It didn't surprise me how popular the hunt had been. I knew it had been the right decision to do it. The numerous photos being uploaded to the website surely vindicated my belief. Just like banning the Chinese from CROUCHING.

I spent the whole night hammering away furiously at the keyboard, thanking people for their support and answering the dozens of e mails. I stopped only to talk to Molly in New York. Our Skype conversation wasn't as straight forward as it would usually have been due to the large number of her pals who wanted to say 'hi' to the head of the CROUCHING community. It was appearing more and more that New York was becoming a hot bed for CROUCHING activity. I must add that they were all a little unsure what to make of midget hunting though. American liberalism gone mad. It would no doubt garner huge support in the deep south mind.

By the time I raided the fridge for the last few pieces of ham it was close to dawn. I glanced at my watch. It said ten past ten. I put on my trainers, grabbed a jacket and left the house in search of a welcome home present for Gemma. The air was cool but not cold and the streets were stealthily quiet. The semi detached houses stood watching me in gloomy silence, waiting for the April sun to wake their sleeping inhabitants. I wandered swiftly but aimlessly looking from side to side for an apt gift. After almost half an hour I finally stumbled on the Holy Grail. "Road works," I said under my breath. Twenty minutes later, covered in sweat but pleased as punch with my efforts, I threw a set of mobile traffic lights onto Gemma's front garden.

Once showered and dressed I went and lay face down on the kitchen floor gripping the big shoe tightly. Even as I admired once more the huge platform sole my thoughts drifted to

Lucy. All I could think about was her and her old man walking hand and hand on a warm moonlit beach and having wild siesta sex sessions. "Am I in love?" I said out loud to the big shoe, half expecting a reply. Dark clouds were gathering and it wasn't good. By the time it was getting close to me leaving for my St Mary's Church CROUCH I could barely lift myself off the floor.

I drank a quick mug of strong coffee and headed off once more; the big shoe tucked under my arm for moral support. The traffic light looked great as it glistened with morning dew. Gemma was going to be chuffed to bits. I checked my mobile about twenty times as I walked slowly towards the church, desperately hoping for a message from Lucy. The only one I got was from Craney saying he'd be at the CROUCH. I was glad to hear from him and wondered if he'd turn up still wearing his nun's gear.

On reaching the church there was cars parked everywhere. You could tell it was Easter, there was never normally anywhere near such a turnout for a Sunday service. The long line of cherry trees, almost in blossom, reminded me I really ought to do a spot of tree climbing soon. The bells rang out the hour of ten and I automatically checked my watch. The thing was fast by ten minutes. However, whatever my timing issues I was surprised to see a sizeable gathering of the community already outside the front doors of the church. Sunday's had almost always been a solo event for me, so seeing twenty members immediately lifted my mood. I shook everyone by the hand and gave Craney a big hug. Surprisingly he wasn't in his habit. Once the greetings were complete I got straight down to business. Seeing as we had such a good turnout I thought I better say a few words, so instead I just bent my knees and slipped into a 160 degree right leg slightly ajar CROUCH. The community CROUCHED in unison beside me and a hush fell over us, respectful of our surroundings. Behind me I heard the church organ grind into action and voices begin to sing a hymn I vaguely recognised.

After a few minutes; a perfectly suitable length of time for an Easter Sunday CROUCH, I stood upright and said, "thank you all for attending today's Easter Sunday CROUCH outside St Mary's Church in Plympton. There will be a further CROUCH today outside Comet at Marsh Mills, high noon. I hope to see you all there."

I chatted to a few members, mostly about the midget hunt and turned down a number of offers for lifts saying I wanted to do a bit of kerb jumping before the next CROUCH. This wasn't exactly true; I was not on the most sociable of moods and knew no one would try to come between me and a good old kerb jump. So I bid my farewells and made my way across the road and into St Mary's park, an old haunt of my 1970's childhood. Memories that should bring a smile to my sullen face in fact only deepened my gloomy outlook of the world. The brief lifting of spirits I had felt when seeing the community outside the church had quickly dissipated and a black mood bore down on me.

The walk to Marsh Mills took longer than I had planned due to the fact that I stopped a number of times to practice a few new CROUCHES along the way. It seemed to help with my mood which was continuing to go up and down quite spectacularly. One minute I felt ready to reach for a rope, the next I felt on top of the world. Whatever was going on in my broken mind it wasn't great either way. Anyhow, I still arrived in plenty of time to meet up with Andy and Craney for a coffee at the MacDonald's opposite the next CROUCHING venue. We sat outside on a small wooden bench and watched as various members of the community arrived. Again, as the numbers swelled and the excited chatter of midget hunts filled the air, I felt my spirits soar only to fall spectacularly again when someone mentioned Lucy. It took Andy to punch me in the arm and tell me it was midday to bring me back to the task in hand and once again I couldn't fail to be impressed by the large turnout. I lost count at thirty five, but there must have been at least a dozen more, many of whom were totally new faces; young faces. I walked slowly to the entrance of the electrical retail outlet, turned and raised an arm before the expectant faces. Craney couldn't resist letting out a loud bark and after a few 'moos' a hush fell. I waited a few more seconds before saying loudly, "today is the first of a week long number of CROUCHES. To celebrate this all animal noises are permitted and any degree of knee bend allowed. I will be performing a lower left leg uplift 150 degree CROUCH." With that I slid down into the said CROUCH and watched the community follow suit. Shoppers stopped and stared in confusion and incredulity, cars horns started to blare as we blocked the road and at least twenty kids rushed across from MacDonald's to join in with the fun. On top of this the animal noises were terrific and for five minutes the car park was total chaos, sounding like a cross between a farmyard and a zoo. There was no doubt about it, this was CROUCHING at its most spectacular and as normal Lenny was busy capturing it all for posterity. In fact I could see dozens of mobile phones being held aloft doing the same thing. I checked my watch; it said ten past ten. Slowly I stood back upright and for the second time that morning I said, "thank you all for attending today's high noon CROUCH outside Comet on Marsh Mills, Plympton. For all of you who are first time CROUCHERS I would like to welcome you all to the CROUCHING community and to ask you all to keep an eye on the CROUCHING In Random Places website for details of tomorrow's and all future CROUCHES. And remember to always measure your children's heads regularly."

After doing the rounds, mainly answering ridiculous questions from students, this time I did accept a lift in big Andy's van to the Josh for a pint. When I entered I was cheered like some returning hero from the war. Everyone wanted to hear about the midget hunt and the latest CROUCHING activity. Many of the students from the Comet CROUCH had turned up and I was in the middle of a conversation about some sort of appearance in the Student Union when I got a tap on the shoulder from a tall thin chap of about my age, sporting a pair of John Lennon like round spectacles.

"Mr Christie?" He said in a neutral tone.

I nodded in response already guessing he was a journalist. I was right. He had that sort of shifty look I would expect to see in a man of that profession. Or was I just imagining it? Anyway, thirty minutes later, sat in the beer garden I had finished telling him my family history warts and all and was happily explaining my problems with the Chinese.

"Of course it's not racist; you do realise that Chinese women have sideways fanny's don't you?"

The chap almost dropped his pen. "I'm sorry?" He spluttered.

"And tiny feet. I'd have to be mad to let them come on one of my CROUCHES. They'd be falling over every time they bent their knees. Imagine the potential for damages? I'd be ruined in weeks." I made a flippant gesture with my hands and went on, "then there's the yellow skin issue. It's like they're taking the piss out of typhoid sufferers."

"Well, er, yes," the journo stuttered. "That's a very interesting point of view."

I spouted on quite happily about my fear of badgers, midgets, plumbers and people with a wandering eye, going into great detail as always about water melon headed children and the need for midget pits. Eventually I shut up and reached for the big shoe which I had put under the bench. I placed it purposefully down in front of the bemused reporter and said loudly, "isn't that the most beautiful thing you have ever seen in your life?"

I went on to explain how important the big shoe had become in my life and how it helped me with my depression. He questioned me at length about my mental health issues and I answered with absolute honesty. For once he nodded along with me and listened intently with none of the raised eyebrows or quizzical expressions. Eventually he looked at his watch and appeared to make a decision. He said, "one last question Mr Christie. What are your plans for the future?"

"How do you mean?"

"Well, in regard to CROUCHING for example?"

"I think I am on the brink of delivering something great to the world," I answered somewhat pompously. "So yes, CROUCHING will no doubt be very much at the forefront of my life over the next few years. Mind you," I added, "I am partial to the odd lean and have recently been researching various things to lean on. You know, pillar boxes, black painted gates, fishmongers windows are just a few examples."

On this piece of fishmonger related information he glanced at his watch again, put his note pad and tiny tape recorder into his jacket pocket and stood up. Offering me his hand he thanked me for his time and left me with a business card in case I needed to get in contact. I watched him leave, drained the remainder of my drink, picked up the big shoe from the bench top and left as well. I needed to be alone. After all the talk I felt empty once more and the last thing I needed was a pub full of drunken well wishers pestering me. I had no idea where I was headed; I just let my legs take me anywhere they wanted.

A few hours later I found myself at the very highest point of Plympton, Dorsmouth Rock and stood looking down at the panoramic view below. Houses, shops, churches, schools, were all laid out beneath me. There it was, my whole life lying far below me. I felt terribly sad. I could feel the old cloud getting closer again, almost overhead in fact. I looked up at the faint blue sky, the sun was still visible but I knew my face was in shadow. I shivered involuntarily and looked around for the icy finger that touched my spine. There was no one there of course. There never was. I was always alone. That's how it always was.

"This is how it is meant to be," I said quietly, clinging tightly to the big shoe. I thought about Lucy and sat down on the cold granite. I could smell her in the cool air and when I closed my eyes I could taste her. Her voice came in gentle waves but my ears could not quite hear what she was saying. I sat there for a long time, lost in a sort of dream and when I finally opened my eyes it was pitch black and I felt like my world had ended such was the waves of depression washing over me. I knew it was coming but I had never felt it hit me so hard before. I was paralysed with despair and self loathing. Some people's depression creeps up on them over a period of months but mine always come like a hammer blow. I knew that I was on the very edge. I no longer wanted to be part of this world. I was lost. All the thoughts and emotions that I kept locked tightly away now emerged en – mass to overwhelm me. My failed marriage, my lost son, my lost youth, my lost health, my lost love. Everything was lost. "I am lost," I heard myself mumble.

It was almost completely dark as I left the rock and made my way down the wonderfully named 'Drunken Bridge Hill.' A car flashed by me almost knocking me into the hedge but I didn't even flinch. I knew where I was heading and nothing was about to get in my way. I walked swiftly through the dark streets, a man on a mission. It took me just over half an hour to get to my destination, another narrow, tree lined dark road, Stoggy Lane. Another good name I thought briefly. It ran parallel to the main London to Penzance railway and it was this that had drawn me like a magnet. At the point where the lane went under the tracks and go steeply uphill I scrambled up the embankment and sat on the bridge wall with a grim smile on my face. I looked down at the dark tracks gripping the big shoe tightly.

After what seemed an eternity I heard the familiar sound of hissing from the railway lines signalling an oncoming train. I calmly placed the big shoe on the grass verge and stepped out purposefully onto the railway line. "This is how it is meant to be," I said quietly as I lay down across the track in the almost total darkness. The noise of the train when it came was immense. I braced myself, heard a blast of a horn, saw bright lights in the corners of my closed eyes and a split second later felt a huge rush of wind against my face as the train rushed past me on the other line. I opened my eyes fully, got slowly up and looking up at the stars shook my head. "Fucking trains," I mumbled, turned around and walked back to the grass verge. I picked up the big shoe and walked home. I spent the rest of the night laying face down on the kitchen floor.

CHAPTER FIFTEEN

RAINDROPS KEEP FALLING ON MY HEAD

CROUCHING Community Membership 7,233

After sending text messages to my son, Gemma and Nikki I found myself in the bathroom staring into the mirror. I needn't have stared as a quick glance would have told me how bad I looked. My hair looked lank and greasy, falling down over my lined forehead. My face looked tired and drawn. I ignored my dishevelled looks and tried to remember where today's CROUCH was taking place. I couldn't even remember if I had posted a venue on the website. I went back downstairs and quickly checked on the computer. Nothing. I looked at my watch, it said ten past ten. I looked at the bottom of the computer screen; the time said 9:24. There must have been some sort of power cut I thought. I was pacing up and down the front room trying to think of a suitable location when my father rang. His tone was somewhat frosty.

"Ah so you're alive then?" He hadn't a clue how apt a question it was.

Our conversation was brief. I was informed that my mental health nurse wanted to see me at my parent's house the following day. I could hear the disappointment in my father's voice; another person to add to the list of people I was letting down. The short conversation left me feeling even more depressed. It did however bring a suitable CROUCHING venue to mind, 4 Maidenwell Road, the place of my birth. I was one of the few true Plymptonians, born at home as opposed to a hospital in Plymouth. I quickly posted the address on the website, hoping that at this late time no one would see it as I wasn't in the mood for company.

I hadn't even begun to digest the railway incident as I now thought of it and as I crossed over the railway on one of those steel foot bridges I was really tempted to just jump off. The railways tracks below seemed to be almost calling me. I must admit this would have been an excellent suicide spot and I found myself mulling over the best ten suicide spots in the area. Eventually I put these thoughts to one side; just in time as I turned into Maidenwell Road. I ambled up the steep hill, one side of which was a long row of terraced houses, the other more modern semi detached. My old house, number 4, was right at the top of the hill on the terraced side. When I lived there back in the 1970's the house was painted a shocking pink but unfortunately now was much the same dull colour as all the others. I was shocked to see seven or eight people mulling around outside, clearly waiting for the head of the CROUCHING community to arrive. I was prepared for a solo CROUCH considering the lateness of my post, yet here they were. I couldn't fault their commitment but it didn't help with my mood whatsoever.

As I greeted them I saw that all but one were students from the university. They were becoming regulars at all the CROUCHES and I recognised a tall spiky haired girl dressed in punky sort of clothes, her white spikes and pink Doc Marten boots making her stand out in a number of my more obscure venue choices of late. However, I could not bring myself to get into any sort of long conversations so I went directly to my old front door and slipped into a rather dull 150 degree double knee bend CROUCH. The others followed suit and soon the only noise to be heard was the singing of a nearby blackbird and the whispers of a few neighbours who had come out to stand in their doorways wondering what on earth was going on in their quiet street. Normally I would have let out a few barks at them but my thoughts remained ones of overwhelming emotion of the blackest kind. I looked around at the young smiling faces and longed to be one of them. For them CROUCHING was a bit of fun; for me it was a matter of life and death. I let them have their fun for five minutes or so before I stood upright and said, "thank you all for attending today's CROUCH outside 4 Maidenwell Road in Plympton. Tomorrow's CROUCH will be at the same time next to the bus shelter on Glen Road, opposite the junction with Parkstone Lane." With that I quickly walked off before anyone had time to converse with me.

I walked for almost eight hours, never breaking my steady pace; constantly checking my phone for a message from Lucy. The only text I received was from Gemma asking how I was feeling. I ignored it. Every few minutes I would look up at the sky, checking for the black cloud which I knew was somewhere up there mocking me. Good old Kirkland, he's such a laugh. That's what everyone said about me...They ought to try walking in my shoes. When I finally got home it was dark and I had no recollection of where I had been apart from stopping at a small shop to buy a drink. The day had passed by in a fog of dark thoughts and sour memories. I drank two mugs of coffee, swallowed a couple of pieces of the old wafer thin and reluctantly switched on the computer.

Five minutes later I was sat in stunned silence as I watched a You Tube video of Molly's latest New York CROUCH. What was advertised as a CROUCH outside some deli had turned into what must be 500 people blocking a whole street. It was breathtaking. Normally I would have spent hours pouring over the video time and time again, looking for Chinese faces amongst the CROUCHERS but I just didn't have it in me. I sent a message of congratulations to Molly, noticing that I had over a hundred e mails most of which looked to be praising my recent efforts. I should be doing celebratory cartwheels such was the momentum the community was gaining but all I could do was go to the kitchen, lay face down on the floor and think about what the fuck I was doing still breathing.

I was still there the following morning and made no effort to tidy myself before heading off to my parents. I didn't even brush my teeth let along put a comb through my hair.

"I can't understand him," my mother was saying to dad. "What's so wrong with midgets?"

"Big heads," I mumbled.

"What?"

"It doesn't matter," I mumbled again.

"Let the nurse sort it out," my dad snapped but mother wasn't satisfied.

"Big heads? Who has big heads?"

"For Christ's sake," dad snapped at her again.

"Well it's ridiculous, dressing up at his age and putting midgets in bags. Where were you going to put the poor things."

"In a midget pit that Craney has dug."

"Oh I might have guessed he'd be involved. I warned you about him didn't I? "She turned to my father and said, "didn't I warn him about that Craney?"

I was just about to tell her that Craney had given me a big shoe when the door bell rang. It wasn't my normal mental health nurse, instead it was a young man called Dave who seemed a bit uneasy all round. I gave him the usual bullshit of saying I was sleeping well, taking all my medication, not drinking etc etc. The good thing about my low mood meant that I answered all his questions calmly and pleasantly and with none of the crazy remarks that would no doubt have only landed me in trouble and maybe hospitalised. I explained the midget hunt as a grave error brought about from drinking heavily on my medication and boys just having a bit of bank holiday fun. I agreed it was a grave error that I would not be making again. The meeting seemed to ease my mother's concerns although my father gave me one of those looks only father's can give as I left the house and made my way to the day's CROUCH.

The bus shelter on Glen Road opposite Parkstone Lane was completely empty when I arrived. A steady drizzle was falling and if ever there was a desolate CROUCHING venue then this was it. I checked my watch; it said ten past ten. I sat down on the metal bench inside the shelter and waited to see if anyone would turn up. I wasn't particularly hopeful as I had made no mention of it on the website. After five minutes a couple of teenagers arrived and I asked them if they were here for the CROUCH. They just looked at me with worried expressions and when a bus arrived shortly after they couldn't get on it quick enough. After a second bus came and went a small red Fiat pulled into the bus stop and two girls got out. I recognised the tall spikey haired one immediately. They were both full of smiles and excitement. I got up to greet them, also recognising the smaller, by some margin, of the two as another regular of recent CROUCHES.

"Hey," said spikey hair. "I'm Annie and this is Jo."

"Hello ladies," I said graciously and shook their hands. "I'm Kirkland Christie, head of the CROUCHING community. I think it's just going to be the three of us today."

"Goody goody," squealed Annie excitedly. "Can I do the bit at the end? The words?"

"I don't see why not," I agreed. Her sheer enthusiasm was irresistible and on top of that both the girls were more than passably attractive which always helped. I went out of the bus stop, the drizzle cold on my skin and wasted no time in saying, "we are gathered here for the high noon CROUCH outside the bus shelter on Glen Road opposite the junction with Parkstone Lane. I will be performing a 140 degree left foot slightly open double knee bend CROUCH." With that I slid down into the said CROUCH and smiled at the two girls as they did the same. Jo smiled back; a sexy looking girl if ever there was one. She had large green eyes and fair hair not quite reaching her shoulders. She couldn't have been much taller than five feet which was a concern but she appeared to be all in proportion, except for a pair of extremely large breasts which were shown off to great effect by a low cut green top. I tried not to stare but it wasn't easy. She gave me the impression she knew I was staring at her tits and she thoroughly enjoyed it. Her broad smile spread wide across her face and she kept glancing towards Annie as if she needed her approval. Annie herself was a totally different kettle of fish altogether. She was easily 5'10 and looked like she has been transported directly from the summer of 1976. A punk chic look that was a breath of fresh air in today's somewhat grey society. Her long legs were on show in all their glory; a short tartan miniskirt, black tights and her customary pink Doc Martens drawing my attention to them. A black leather jacket, studded dog collar and Annie Lennox like hair finished off the look. I found myself looking at her fascinated and wondered how my hair would look bleached white. I turned back to Jo who caught me staring at her and winked a green eye and I suddenly found myself wishing I was 21 again. Another wave of depression hit me and I was glad when Annie coughed loudly and did her bit.

"Ladies and gentlemen, thank you for attending today's CROUCH outside a bus stop on Glen Road in Plympton." She looked at me for help but I remained impassive. "Oh," she suddenly blurted out. "And don't forget to measure all your children's heads and have a look under your bed each day." She laughed. "That was crap wasn't it?"

I nodded. "Total shit."

"I thought she did okay," offered Jo. "Much better than I would have."

"Sorry girls, I'm not in the best of moods."

Annie came up to me, she smelt good. "You didn't seem your normal crazy self yesterday Mr CROUCHER." She really was quite striking.

"Can we do anything to help?" Offered Jo.

"It's not been a good few days for me," I admitted. "You know, the old black clouds and all that."

"Depression?" Asked Jo.

"Of the very darkest kind," I answered honestly.

Annie took hold of my arm and said, "okay Mr CROUCHER, why don't we go and get a coffee somewhere and you can tell me and Jo all about it."

Ten minutes later the three of us were sat in Chaplin's cafe; not the most salubrious of venues, being a builders merchant, but it did have the advantage of being just off Strode Road, the home of Hall Graves and Lee. Annie had made Jo drive past it twice and had been desperate to get out and CROUCH but I was having none of it.

"You know we are both studying to become doctors," said Jo as she placed the tray with three mugs of coffee on it down on the table.

"I'm the general practice one," added Annie, "and Jo here is the psychologist one."

"Fuck me, you lot are everywhere," I said quietly, then added, "sorry, I have had my fair share of shrinks and the like lately."

We chatted about their courses for a while. When I say *we* chatted, what I mean is they did. I just sat in a sort of numbed silence, nodding now and again to look interested. Annie could see I was not right and after a while stretched out a long slender hand and touched mine gently. "Is there anything we can do to help? You can tell us anything you want or nothing at all, it doesn't matter. You just look so sad."

I looked at her for a few seconds. She really was striking. A pale face with high cheek bones, emphasised by contrasting bright red lips. Her blue eyes sparkled with intelligence and the white cropped hair gave an edge of danger. "It's been a bad few days," I said, not wanting to give anything of myself away to these two strangers. Yet a few minutes later I found myself totally outpouring what had happened to me since Lucy had gone. The two girls sat in silence as I told them of my suicide attempt and how I felt it was only a matter of time before I got the right track and finished the job properly. When I had finished my tale of woe Annie got up and came around to my chair and hugged me tightly.

"Oh you poor thing Mr CROUCHER."

"It is what it is," I said back, not returning the embrace.

"Nonsense," replied Annie as she broke free of and stood looking down at me. "I am not having any of that. I'll drag you to the doctor if need be."

Jo joined in. "I can drive you to the doctor's right now if you want. We can come in with you if it helps."

I shook my head. "I have had more than enough of all the quacks and their underlings."

We argued a bit more before both the girls realised I wasn't about to hand myself over to the white coat brigade, or start taking my medication either. I attempted to describe my depression but didn't make a good job of it. Annie though, seemed to understand and went about telling me how much pleasure I gave to loads of people and what a one off character I was. "You are the head of the CROUCHING community and we all love you," she said before finally sitting back down.

"I could do with someone like you when I'm laying face down on the kitchen floor," I said finally raising a brief smile.

"It would be like all my dreams come true," laughed Annie.

"A ten hour stint of lino sniffing isn't much fun."

"I wouldn't care whatsoever, if it meant you kept away from the train lines."

An idea came into my head, one that I had mulled over for some time but which I had recently put to the back of my thoughts as the midget hunt had come to the fore. "There is something you could do for me," I said slowly.

Annie raised her eyebrows and replied mischievously, "I knew it."

I grunted and said, "it's nothing like that. I've been thinking about organising a one off huge CROUCH. A Mayday CROUCH. A worldwide CROUCHING event that captures the imagination and grabs the headlines like the midget hunt did. I want people all over the world to CROUCH as one and with us lot in Plymouth leading the way. I want banners up everywhere, covering the city and graffiti sprayed everywhere announcing the CROUCHING community. All sorts of stuff so that everyone knows about it. I am going to bombard the press promoting it. I want thousands involved. You can help massively with the student population here."

"That's more like the Mr CROUCHER we know. We'd love to help wouldn't we Jo?" Jo nodded and smiled broadly. I tried not to look at her tits.

I went on, "I reckon you could draw in hundreds of students. Mind you, no Chinese. That goes without saying. If they can get 500 odd students in New York CROUCHING without much effort imagine what we can do if we really go to town on it. A thousand? Two thousand? We can bring the city centre to a grinding halt."

"Wouldn't we do it in Plympton?" Jo asked; a very good point.

"No, it would have to be somewhere in the city centre in order to gain maximum publicity. I hate the thought of CROUCHING outside of my comfort zone but in this instance there is no choice."

We talked for another half hour about the viability of a Mayday CROUCH. I bought another round of coffees and for the first time in days felt something close to my old self. The two young students' enthusiasm was totally genuine and lifted my spirits. When I finally got up to go Jo offered me a lift but I turned her down. "I like to walk. I look out for bushes to hide in and kerbs to jump off." I stretched out a hand and shook Annie's first, then Jo's and said solemnly, "the head of the CROUCHING community would like to thank it's younger members for all their support during these tough times." With that I wrote down my mobile number which Annie had asked for and left the cafe not looking back. I went out into the rain and tried to figure out what sort of mood I was in.

By the time I reached Gemma's I was soaked through; the fine drizzle doing the same job as a typhoon. Thankfully there was no sign of Gemma and the girls so I went about having a shower, brushing my teeth and generally trying to make myself look reasonably presentable. I couldn't bring myself to shave and when I stared at myself in the mirror I was shocked to see how drawn and tired I looked. The beard growth only added to my dishevelled appearance. I considered eating but my appetite was non existent. I settled for a chunk of fruit cake and ate it staring out of the kitchen window thinking about Lucy. Eventually I dragged myself away from the gloomy landscape and went and turned on the computer. I posted:

I would like to thank all of you who attended today's CROUCH outside the bus shelter on Glen Road opposite the junction with Parkstone Lane. A special thank you goes out to Jo and Annie of Plymouth University for helping me open a door when all of them appeared closed.

Kirkland Christie   Head of the CROUCHING Community

It was an unusual post for me to make but then I was in an unusual mood. I forced myself
to go through a dozen or so e mails and sat for a couple of hours replying meticulously to
each one as well as offering a couple of quotes to some journalists who had shown more
than a bit of interest in the community. There were still a few messages of abuse from
midgets and midget fanciers including one which said he was the second hardest dwarf in
Cornwall and he was coming for me. That cheered me up a little. I replied to the message
asking him to send me his head measurements to see if I needed to take the threat seriously.
Just before I hit the kitchen floor I made one final tweet:

No matter how many hours are spent lying face down on the kitchen floor I cannot shake
this feeling of guilt. It all started when I ate a spring roll...

I was still on the kitchen floor when Nikki arrived with some bread and milk for Gemma.
"I guessed you would be lying there," she said laughing.

"It's no laughing matter Nikki," I replied without moving. "I am trying to decide where to
hold a Mayday CROUCH. It's going to be spectacular."

"Ah, right. I should have guessed. Any news from Lucy?"

"Nothing whatsoever."

"She probably left her mobile at home, you know, worried that you might ring her in the
middle of the night. Anyway it's only a few days now and she'll be back."

I let out a sigh, and still not looking up at Nikki said, "she's probably getting her wedding
fucking vows renewed."

Nikki did her best to reassure me but it was all to no avail. Just the thought of Lucy and
her husband together had sunk me down into the depths once more. I laid glumly sniffing

the lino and just let out a grunt when Nikki asked if I wanted a coffee. She had just placed the mug on the floor beside me when I let out a loud shout of, "Clive's Tackle!"

"What?" Nikki exclaimed spilling her own drink some of which splashed down on the lino next to me.

"Clive's Tackle shop. For the May Day CROUCH."

"Christ I wondered what the hell you were on about."

"Keep up woman," I said finally getting up off the floor as I warmed to my subject. "Or Devon Pine Furniture on Exeter Street."

"Kirk, forget about CROUCHING for a minute. How are you feeling? You look awful."

"Thanks. You should have seen me a few hours ago before I showered. I don't think I have brushed my teeth in days. By the way what *day* is it?" I really had no idea.

Nikki laughed. "It's Tuesday you nutter."

"Oh right," I mumbled not really caring one way or the other.

"You're famous you know Kirk. I can't go anywhere without people asking about you."

"Yet I feel like shit."

"You'll be fine. Only a few more days to wait. And Gemma will be home in a minute."

"What about the Conservative Club on Mutley Plain?"

"What about it?"

"For the May Day CROUCH Nikki. Keep up."

Before Nikki could reply we saw Gemma's car pull up outside. The girls were out of the back doors practically before the car stopped but were halted in their tracks by Gemma's booming voice telling them in no uncertain terms to take some bags in with them.

"Yikes, she sounds happy," whispered Nikki as I followed her out into the drizzle to offer Gemma a hand.

"I need a seriously large fucking drink," barked Gemma as she opened the boot. She was just about to greet us properly when the girls gave out a squeal of delight as they set their eyes on the traffic light for the first time.

"Oh for fuck's sake Kirk," said Gemma, obviously unimpressed by my latest gift and swept past me almost knocking me over with a huge bag. Nikki raised her eyebrows at me and I just shrugged and went a grabbed a suitcase.

For the next hour the house was in total chaos. Gemma screamed hysterically at the girls, who in turn screamed back and Nikki ran about trying to help out but only made things worse. I slunk off to my bedroom and sat on the bed holding the big shoe. I didn't go back downstairs until an Indian Takeaway arrived and Gemma forced me to show her some of the video footage from the midget hunt. The rest of the evening was spent watching the women of the house almost wet themselves in hysterics as they sat crowded around the computer screen. It was only when Nikki had left and the girls had gone to bed that Gemma turned to the subject of Lucy.

"It's been a tough few days Gem," I admitted honestly. "Lucy's part of it. Most of it. Then there's Zak, the sausage kings, the Chinese...Everything is a struggle."

Gemma walked over and put her arms around me. "You've missed your auntie Gem haven't you?"

I nodded. "I have actually. I've spent an awful lot of time on the kitchen floor."

"How's the big shoe?"

"Truly beautiful Gem."

I knew I had to tell her about the 'railway incident' and struggled to find the right words. Eventually I broke free from her embrace and looked into her bright green eyes, a serious expression on my face.

"What's happened Kirk?" Gemma could sense trouble.

"I had a kind of episode." I was struggling to find the right words.

"What do you mean?"

I gulped and said, "a suicidal sort of episode." It was obvious from her reaction that she hadn't been expecting this. I told her everything. When I had finished Gemma had tears rolling down her cheeks.

"Oh Kirk, you silly fucking fool. What would we have all done without you? We all love you." She wiped her eyes then added, "fucking hell mate, I'm never leaving you on your own ever again."

"Don't be ridiculous Gem, you know how my brain works."

"I mean it. I should have seen this coming." She rubbed her hands together trying to get a grip on the situation. "And what about now Kirk? Are you still feeling that way?"

I smiled and replied, "let's just say that the train drivers of the Great Western Railway can go to work without worrying about me."

Gemma didn't respond to my light hearted remark and instead got up and disappeared into the kitchen. After a few minutes when she hadn't returned I went in after her only to find her standing smoking at the back door. The drizzle still fell and the breeze was enough that she was getting steadily wetter by the second.

"Gem, it's okay, honestly," I said earnestly.

She turned to look at me, her cheeks now covered in streams of black mascara. "But it's not Kirk is it? Look at you. You look like someone who's given up on life. I can see it in your expression; in your eyes."

"I'll be fine Gem," I said trying to reassure both her and myself.

"Obviously you fucking won't," she snapped.

"I'm sure it will pass soon," I offered.

"Well you are staying in my shadow until it does and no fucking arguing."

I nodded slowly then added, "I still have CROUCHING commitments every day this week."

"Then either me or Nikki will go with you. Thankfully the schools are still off."

"Fucking schools," I said quietly but loud enough for Gemma to hear.

"Oi! You ought to be thrilled to have two gorgeous guardian angels looking out for you."

"I Know. And I am. I just don't like putting you out that's all."

Gemma burst into laughter. "Mate, you've been putting me out ever since I first clamped my eyes on you."

"I tell you what? You can take the big shoe to bed with you as a thank you."

"Fuck off," Gemma laughed. "That's more like the old Kirkland."

CHAPTER SIXTEEN

RAPID CYCLING BUT NOT THE TOUR DE FRANCE KIND

CROUCHING Community Membership 8,437

The head of the CROUCHING community is pleased to announce the first ever world wide May Day CROUCH. At high noon on Sunday 1st May there will be a CROUCH in unison across all four corners of the globe (except China for obvious reasons) in honour of nothing other than the right to bend one's knees in any old random venue. Start making plans my friends as this is going to be the most important knee bending fiesta since I took my first foray into the world of CROUCHING, outside Hall Graves and Lee many years ago.

Kirkland Christie   Head of the CROUCHING Community

Lord knows how long I had spent hammering away at the computer but when I finally called it a night I was drained and exhausted. I stumbled to my bed and fell asleep almost immediately. When Gemma shook me and handed me a coffee I felt like I had been sleeping for days, not just a few hours.

  "How are you feeling?" Gemma asked sitting on the bed next to me and slurping at a steaming mug of tea.

"Randy," I answered with my standard reply.

"Fuck me, you must be ill," Gemma laughed. "Anyway, I'm glad you slept as *I* tossed and turned all night."

"You should have taken me up on the big shoe offer."

"Yeah right. Seriously, how are you feeling today?"

"I'm fine Gem, honestly." She didn't look at all reassured but left me to drink my coffee in peace. I finally felt able to manage a shave and looked a lot more like my old self by the time I went downstairs. "Don't forget the high noon CROUCH," I reminded Gemma who was in the kitchen surrounded by huge piles of washing.

"I know!" She exclaimed, at the same time my mobile began to buzz. I didn't recognize the number so I let it ring through to voicemail. I then became worried that it might have been Lucy using a different phone. I quickly dialled the number to retrieve the message.

"Hi, Mr CROUCHER. It's Annie from yesterday. You haven't said where today's CROUCH is. I hope you're okay."

I considered ringing her back but instead did a bit of hoovering and dishwashing much to Gemma's pleasure. At 11:45, according to Gemma; I made it ten past ten, we got in the car and headed off for the day's high noon CROUCH. The girls were beside themselves with excitement at the thought of witnessing a CROUCH in the flesh and were a bit confused when I instructed their mother to pull up next to a pillar box on Wolverwood Lane, Plympton.

"Where is everyone?" One of the girls shouted as I got out of the car and into a driving wind complete with pouring rain.

"This is everyone," I shouted back to them as I slammed the car door shut and stepped beside the pillar box. As I bent down into a 150 degree double knee bend left foot slightly raised CROUCH, I smiled at the girls as they stared somewhat incredulously at me. This was definitely not what they were expecting. I cut a sad, lonely figure as I CROUCHED alone in the driving rain. Water poured down over my dark glasses which looked totally foreign in such an environment and to add to my downcast mood a bus went by and sprayed me with rain water from the road. I was just coming to the end of what I reckoned was five minutes when a car drove past and someone shouted 'wierdo!' out of the window at me. Probably, I thought and walked back to the car.

"Is that it?" Cried the girls in unison.

"Yep that's it," I replied.

Gemma looked at me with a concerned expression. "Are you alright mate?"

I nodded but said nothing. In fact I didn't say anything until my phone rang just as we arrived home. It was Craney.

"You're fucking famous mate," he half screamed into my ear. "Have you seen the paper?"

"Shit, I'd forgotten all about that mate. Is it bad?" It was true, I had completely forgotten about my interview in the pub beer garden.

"It's fucking brilliant," Craney ranted. "They've depicted you as some madman running an underground cult. The headline says 'unhinged' and there's a photo of you in the sheriff gear. There's a great one of all of us outside the pub. Here listen to this," I heard the rustle of paper. "Plymouth is at the centre of a terrifying new craze in which midgets have been victimised and subject to foul abuse by gangs of men, most of whom are in their forties. This culminated with the so called Good Friday Midget Hunt in which the leader Kirkland Christie and many of his followers were arrested. It's fucking brilliant matey."

"It's an absolute travesty," I replied feeling the blood rise to my cheeks.

Craney wouldn't be put off though. "It says that Mr Christie, a bi polar sufferer who is currently under the care of the Plymouth Community Mental Health Team, claims that midgets are evil due to them having heads the size of water melons and extremely short arms." He stopped reading due to laughing but after a few seconds went on, "Christie, who claims his full time occupation is crouching, no capitals by the way, and refers to himself as the head of the crouching community, states that there are thousands of members across the world and that the group's headquarters is at a local M.O.T. centre, Hall Graves and Lee on Strode Road, Plympton. One of the employees there says he often sees Christie crouching outside at various times of the day."

I wasn't having any of that and I shouted down the phone, "I always CROUCH at ten past fucking ten!"

"There's plenty more," said Craney excitedly, obviously enjoying being the purveyor of such dramatic news, but I told him I'd heard all I wanted to hear. Indeed I heard nothing but the headlines as my phone rang constantly for the rest of the day. One of the calls turned out to be from Annie.

"Hey Mr CROUCHER, how are you? I take it you have seen the headlines?"

"It's a fucking outrageous piece of liberal propaganda. The midget fancying press at their absolute worse."

"You've become quite the celebrity," she laughed.

"If you say so."

"Too much of a star to tell me where today's CROUCH was?"

"Oh yeah. Sorry, I wanted to CROUCH alone. And besides, it was pissing down."

"I have a big umbrella which you could have shared. When nothing was posted on the website I got really worried. And then when I heard you were in the newspaper I shit myself." She did actually sound concerned.

"I'm fine Annie. Not jumping over the moon but not jumping off a bridge either. Although Craney telling me that CROUCHING was written in small letters did nearly push me over the edge. Fucking liberty." I could feel the blood rushing to my head in anger. "So, as my right hand woman what do you intend to do about it?"

"I like that. Your right hand woman. I could find out where he lives and organise a big rave in his front garden." We both laughed. Talking of organising, have you decided on a venue for the May Day extravaganza?"

"Indeed I have. Outside the Devonshire Pine furniture shop on Exeter Street. Nice and close to you lot and a great place to bring the bank holiday traffic to a stand still." It was a good venue; right on the main road into Plymouth's shopping centre and waterfront and also in the heart of student land.

"I love it. It's perfect. I will be able to drag loads of students there. Right what about tomorrow's CROUCH?" She was keen, I'll give her that.

"Um..." I stuttered, before saying, "there's a gap in the terrace houses on Underwood Road, around about number 47. It's a passage way through to a back garden. You can't mistake it."

Annie laughed. "You're so funny Mr CROUCHER."

"Yeah, I'm fucking hilarious," I replied sarcastically and hung up.

An hour later I was sat with Nikki and Gemma, the enormity of my new found infamy sinking in. "The ex wife is bound to show Zak," I said with my head in my hands.

"And there's no way your parents won't see it. Or your mental health nurse for that matter," added Nikki for good measure.

"You've really gone and shot yourself in the fucking foot this time mate," said Gemma, pointing out the obvious.

"Fucking midget fanciers the lot of them," I said, my head still in my hands, before lifting it up to stare at Gemma. "I am the fucking law!" I bellowed, making both the women jump and the girls to come running down from upstairs to see what was going on.

"Christ he's off again," laughed Nikki. She was right, I wasn't a happy bunny and that night I banged away at the computer feverishly complaining about everything from the gutter press to a lack of dead badgers on the roads these days. One thing that all the press did bring in though was interest to my world. The CROUCHING community had never been in such rude health and the membership numbers were rapidly approaching 10,000. It appeared that the more outrageous I was the more people seemed to want to join in. At some point during the night I stopped the chat room rants and made the following post:

The head of the CROUCHING community is pleased to announce the May Day CROUCH which will take place outside Devon Pine Furniture Store on Exeter Street, Plymouth at midday on Sunday 1st May. The May Day CROUCH is to be the community's first ever unified CROUCH with members CROUCHING at high noon in their various time zones around the world. I want you all to take part in a worldwide extravaganza of CROUCHING which will bring attention to our wonderful knee bending cause. Get the press involved, the kids involved, your grannies involved. Get everyone involved, except the Chinese of course. Keep checking the web site for updates and let me know what you have planned.

Tomorrow's high noon CROUCH will be outside the narrow gap in the terrace houses somewhere around about number 47 Underwood Road, Plympton. You can't miss it. Unfortunately on this occasion I am going to have to say that no Chinese are permitted to take part.

Kirkland Christie   Head of the CROUCHING Community

I had no idea how long I had been hammering away at the keyboard; I looked at my watch and it said ten past ten. I got up and put the big shoe on as best I could. Ten minutes later Gemma burst into the lounge in her dressing gown to be greeted with the sight of me half running in a circle chanting, "You're the one who fucked my daughter, sucked her tits for an hour and a quarter," over and over extremely loudly.

"Kirk do you know what time it is?" Gemma had to scream to be heard; or she may have just been screaming.

"Yeah, it's ten past ten." I answered without slowing down.

"Try five o fucking clock!"

"You're the one," I poked a finger at her, "who punched my granny, stuck your fist right up her fanny."

"What the hell are you on about?" Gemma looked like she was about to burst.

"Your the one..."

"Shut the fuck up will you!" This time she left me in no doubt she wasn't enjoying my song. "It's way too early for all this shit."

"Gem you don't understand. CROUCHING is the key. It's always been about CROUCHING."

"Great. Now will you please shut the fuck up?"

"Okay. I'm going to get some ham."

"Well do it fucking quietly," Gem snapped before heading back upstairs.

When she came back down a few hours later I was pacing around minus the big shoe and donning a black panama hat that had been sitting on top of the wardrobe in my bedroom since I moved in.

"What's with my uncle's hat?" Gemma asked, still looking a bit pissed off with me. "And all the black get up?" I was dressed head to toe in black.

"I just fancied a change."

"Very mysterious."

"That's what I thought, you know, especially now I am infamous." I grinned at her.

Gemma shook her head. "So where's the CROUCH today then? Somewhere nice?"

I nodded. "Absolutely. It's outside a gap in the terrace houses on Underwood Road. There's a path going through to the back. You know, it splits the terrace."

She shook her head again. "You don't half come up with some shit mate."

This time it was me who shook my head. "It's an obvious choice Gem."

To be honest I wasn't expecting much of a turnout for the CROUCH; the rain was still coming down and Underwood Road was about the worst street in Plympton to try and park on. So I was understandably thrilled and somewhat surprised to see at least twenty people milling around on the narrow pavement. The 'gap' between the houses was already blocked by what looked like students and I could see a lot of these were first time CROUCHERS. The girls were going mad in the back of the car as Gemma pulled over to let me out; they were desperate to join the crowd but their mother was having none of it. I agreed to meet her on pain of death at the local co-op in thirty minutes time.

As more CROUCHERS arrived the always hard to navigate narrow street was being thrown into total chaos. Cars backed up both ways; horns blared; community members spilling out across the road. I watched as curious neighbours peered from windows or came out of their houses to see what all the fuss was about. I saw Annie standing by the gap, her white spiky hair standing out like a beacon. She caught my eye and smiled; her bright ruby red lips parting to reveal perfect white teeth. She was quite a site dressed in tight red shorts with fishnet tights and her pink Doc Marten boots. A short crop top under her leather jacket showed off a tattoo of something across her stomach and today she had a different dog collar around her neck. This one was pink with nasty looking needles sticking out of it. Even with my lovely black hat I felt under dressed beside her.

"Hey Mr CROUCHER," she said and kissed me lightly on the cheek. She smelt of sandalwood or something like that. "I love the black get up; very goth." She grabbed hold of Jo who was slurping at a cardboard cup of something. "We shook a few buddies out of bed didn't we Jo?"

Jo nodded and looked up at me smiling. I was really concerned about her height but her eyes were so green and her smile so innocent that I didn't have the heart to demand a head measuring session. Plus she had her breasts on display again in a ridiculously low cut blouse of some description. In all fairness being between me and Annie probably didn't help in the scheme of things. "You've worked wonders ladies. I don't recognise half the faces here."

"We've already started hammering home the May Day CROUCH," said Jo. "There's going to be loads coming." Her face was flushed with a young exuberance that I found rather touching. A couple of minutes later after I had say a few hello's namely to Lenny and his cousin little Beefy, I removed my hat and held it aloft waiting for calm and quiet.

"Welcome to today's CROUCH outside the gap between 45 and 47 Underwood Road in Plympton. It is good to see many new faces and for those of you who are partaking in your first CROUCH enjoy it and come again. The community grows stronger everyday as more people around the world see the benefits of bending their knees in some random place. Today I will be performing a 120 degree left leg extension CROUCH." And with that I slipped finely into the said position. I stared solemnly ahead and ignored the few nervous giggles of the first timers and it wasn't long before a silence fell over us. I hadn't counted but there must have been between forty and fifty of us. For a few minutes even the cars stopped honking at us and I swear just for a second the sun poked out from behind the heavy grey clouds. After about five minutes I stood upright and watched the community follow suit. I waited for thirty seconds before saying loudly, "thank you all for attending today's high noon CROUCH outside the gap between 45 and 47 Underwood Road, Plympton. Tomorrow there will be a very special midday CROUCH inside Lloyds bank on The Ridgeway, Plympton, in protest of our fellow member Steven Crane being refused an overdraft last week which meant he couldn't buy any drugs for the weekend. I look forward to seeing you all there and please remember to always measure your children's heads at least once a week."

Twenty minutes later I was helping Gemma put the shopping in the boot of the car and telling her how I'd been asked out that evening by one of the students. "Good for you; is she desperate?" I couldn't tell is she was being serious or not so I ignored the jibe and said, "she wishes to honour the head of the CROUCHING community."

"Oh fuck off."

"Anyway I said no. My days of 'piggy back pub crawls' are long past."

"It sounds a blast."

"It sounds like hell, even if she does have big knockers. And besides, there's the Chlamydia issue to consider."

Gemma stopped what she was doing and looked at me. "The what?"

"The Chlamydia issue," I repeated. "All students have it don't they?"

Before Gemma could reply my phone began to buzz. The screen was showing it was a private number; I felt a surge of excitement that it might be Lucy. It wasn't.

"Hello is that Mr Christie?" A female voice I wasn't familiar with.

"Yes, who is this?" I answered curtly.

"Hi," the voice said breezily. "My name's Emma Brooke, I am a freelance journalist. I wondered if you'd be prepared to give me a few minutes of your time?"

I was just about to tell her to 'fuck off' when I stopped myself. "Certainly, come to Lloyds bank on The Ridgeway, Plympton tomorrow at midday. Oh and bring a camera." I hung up smiling. Craney would have his day in the limelight.

I was back on the subject of Chlamydia and whether you could catch it through anal sex when Nikki pulled up next to us. She had arranged to meet Gemma for a beer so I took the opportunity to escape for an hour and headed off to the library. I needed to get on line and start generating interest in Craney's protest CROUCH as soon as possible. The library itself was a temporary one just up the road from where we would be CROUCHING the following day. Someone had burnt the old one down; not before time in my mind. For once there was no mother and toddler groups trashing the place and I smiled at the two women at the counter and headed over to the computers. I could feel their eyes burning in my back as I sat down at a terminal. I had a bit of history with the library; I once demanded they remove all books relating to Chinese cooking and to put the books on Chinese porcelain on the top shelf so that children wouldn't be exposed to such horrors. Today I behaved impeccably and spent half an hour posting on Facebook, Tweeting, messaging and updating the web site the fact that everyone was required for tomorrow's protest CROUCH.

I smiled again at the librarians as I left; no doubt they felt relieved and headed back to find Gemma and Nikki. However, as I reached the pub I could see Nikki ordering another round of drinks so not wanted to join them I walked the short distance to Harewood House and found a nice hedge to hide in. I tried not to bark as an elderly woman passed by and was holding a hand over my mouth when the phone buzzed again. It was Gemma.

"Where are you?"

"Hiding in a bush," I replied as if it was the most normal thing in the world.

"What are you hiding from?" Gemma laughed.

"I'm not sure, fishmongers?"

"Fuck me you're ridiculous. Hurry up I'm waiting on you."

A couple of minutes later I was getting a bollocking from her for making a mess on the car seat. "It's bushage," I said, "it goes with the territory."

"It's a fucking mess is what it is. Fucking bushage. The bollocks you come out with."

With that the girls, who had been stroking a dog tied up outside the Co-op climbed in the back and immediately wanted to know what had been going on.

"Have you been hiding in a bush again Kirk? Can you show us which one it was?"

Gemma was having none of it. "Don't encourage him girls."

I kept my mouth shut during the drive home and mulled over the upcoming days. Lucy was home tomorrow, Zak was home on Sunday and the sausage kings will be back shortly after. I took a long deep breath and tried to gather myself. My mood swings were becoming increasingly erratic and definitely more extreme and I pondered on which way I would go next. A message on the home answer phone from my mother saying she had seen the newspaper didn't help but I tried to remain calm and focused on the return of Lucy. I was subdued all evening, hardly saying a word to Gemma who spent most of the night chatting crap on the phone. I spent an hour on the computer but my heart wasn't really in it and I was just going up to bed when a text came through. I instantly thought of Lucy but it was actually a picture message from Annie, looking resplendent in the hottest pair of hot pants imaginable. Someone had taken a photo of her CROUCHING, her arse cheeks on clear view. The caption said, 'don't you wish you'd come Mr CROUCHER?' I smiled, went to bed and dreamt of talking conger eels...strange.

I arrived outside Lloyds bank the following morning to be greeted by at least fifty members of the community, even though I was pretty early. Very early when I checked my watch. More people were arriving by the minute and I was already in no doubt that this was going to be a special CROUCH. I heard a load of laughter behind me and turned to see Craney wearing a sandwich board that he had somehow 'acquired.' Childlike block capitals of red paint proclaimed, 'give me an overdraft' and he turned to show me the reverse. It read, 'I need DRUGS!'

"Ah good morning Craney, I see you are ready to reapply for some credit."

Craney grinned; he hadn't put his false teeth in, "everyone's come out to help old Craney." He looked absolutely thrilled and indeed he should be as more and more CROUCHERS arrived. I noticed that there was a good turnout of many of the founder members. I could see Lenny stood on a bench, video in hand getting himself ready; Carter was behind him making horrible noises with his trombone, which he had somehow managed to retrieve after the midget hunt arrests. I was about to go over to him but Craney was grabbing hold of me ranting about 'all the young birds who had come out to support him.' He nearly collapsed when Annie appeared beside him and put her arms around him, saying, "we are all behind you."

"Hi Annie," I said casually and introduced her to Craney, who shook her hand and said loudly, "hello I'm Craney. Do you have a boyfriend?"

"Roll your tongue in Craney," I said as Annie laughed. "She's loyal to the head of the CROUCHING community." I turned to look at her and added, "thanks for the picture by the way." This remark sent Craney into a frenzy; Annie noticing his expression said somewhat mischievously, "he's right you know. I do exactly what he tells me."

Craney instantly turned to me and blurted out, "Kirk, can you tell her to do things to me?"

I shook my head and smiled. "Sorry Craney, she only likes chicks." This was probably the worst thing I could have said to him so I tried to change the subject before he passed out. Just at the right moment the journalist who I had spoken to the day before appeared next to us and quickly introduced herself. I gently pushed her in the direction of Craney and briefly explained what we were doing. Craney seemed more than happy at the arrival of another young woman, particularly now that he had her unbridled attention. I managed to swiftly move amongst the community, greeting old friends and shaking the hands of new faces. Still more CROUCHERS arrived. Lenny shouted across the throng to me saying it was almost midday and I quickly joined him on the bench. As I looked around at the expectant faces looking up at me, I realised we must be over 100 strong.

"Good morning members of the CROUCHING community," I said almost shouting but not quite. "We are gathered here today outside Lloyds bank on The Ridgeway, Plympton for a very special CROUCH. Today for the first time ever we will be CROUCHING inside the venue. For those of you who don't know why, it is in protest at the bank's decision to turn down our fellow member Craney's request for an overdraft." A round of, "he needs drugs," calls came from various parts of the crowd and I waited for silence before I went on. "In a few minutes me and Craney will enter the bank alone and then exactly three minutes later big Andy will lead the rest of you in." I gestured towards big Andy. "I want you all to enter in total silence and Dan, you will be the last one in." Dan nodded sombrely. "Once I see Dan I will remove my hat and at that point we will all CROUCH." I jumped down off the bench, pulled Craney away from the young reporter, who already looked like she had the scoop of the month and walked purposefully into Lloyds bank.

We immediately drew laughter from the half dozen queuing customers as well as a couple of smiles from the girls behind the counter. My immediate concern was how on earth we were going to get everyone inside. We joined the queue and it took less than thirty seconds for an officious looking woman to appear and ask us to leave.

"I'm the head of the CROUCHING community and I am here to ask you to reconsider our member Steven Crane's overdraft application." I gestured toward Craney who offered a toothless smile and pointed at his sandwich board.

"I'm sorry but I really am going to have to ask you to leave." The woman was polite but firm.

"But he needs money to buy drugs," I said calmly.

"Not crack," blurted out Craney. "Just a bit of skunk and maybe a couple of E's."

The woman had obviously heard enough and turned on her heels and was buzzed back through the door beside the counter, no doubt to summon reinforcements. Dead on cue big Andy strode purposefully in and within seconds the bank began to fill. I stood watching impassively as faces both familiar and unfamiliar smiled at me as they found their spot to CROUCH. I noticed Annie bossing around a load of students, trying to ensure they all had enough room. Carter came in with the journalist; she had a slightly pained look on her face which was probably from Carter being continuously smutty. She did however quickly perk up as she observed the unfolding scene. Eventually after what felt like an eternity I saw Dan come through the entrance, he had to wave his arms in the air to be able to be seen such was the heaving mass of bodies between us. We were crammed in like sardines. I took no time in removing my hat and holding it in the air.

"We are gathered here today to protest, by way of a one off special CROUCH, the refusal by Lloyds bank on The Ridgeway, Plympton, to give Craney an overdraft, thus stopping him being able to buy any drugs for the weekend." I lowered my arm and slipped easily into a 140 degree right leg slightly ajar CROUCH. Even by my high standards it was a corker. As one the community followed suit and for sixty seconds all that could be heard was the anxious mutterings of the half dozen customers who looked genuinely confused. Then the door by the counter buzzed again and the woman appeared once more this time accompanied by a balding middle aged man; no doubt the manager.

"Okay ladies and gentleman you've made your point, I must insist you all leave the premises now or I will be forced to call the police." Nobody moved an inch.

I was aware of dozens of pairs of eyes on me waiting to see what my response would be. I tried to focus but my mind continuously wandered to Lucy and the fact that she was on her way home. It was Lenny who made me focus on the task at hand as he dropped his video recorder and swore loudly, bringing about a burst of laughter from the CROUCHERS. I caught Annie's eye and she raised her eyebrows in almost a challenge for me to get to grips with the current situation. As I was looking at Annie the bank manager had pushed his way through to Craney, in the presumption that he was the main ringleader. I waited to see what the outcome would be, whilst at the same time considering what chaos we could cause in various retail outlets with numbers like this. I immediately thought of my sworn enemy up the road in Peacocks. Just then Craney let out a deafening 'moo' in the bank manager's face and this was the trigger for a number of 'midget fancier' shouts. I took this as an opportune moment to stand upright before chaos reigned and I shouted, "thank you all for attending today's high noon CROUCH inside Lloyds bank on The Ridgeway, Plympton, to protest about Craney's overdraft refusal."

At this point Craney screamed manically, "I need crack!" I ignored him and went on, "tomorrow will be the last high noon CROUCH and will take place outside Mary Chang's

Chinese Takeaway on Stone Barton Road, Plympton. And remember; always measure your children's heads on a regular basis."

The bank manager, who had wisely backed away from Craney watched more in astonishment than relief as the community left his bank as quickly as they had entered. After just a few minutes it was once more just me and Craney remaining. I walked over the bank manager and looked him straight in the eye. "I can do this everyday for a month if you like."

He didn't look impressed but remained calm. "Gentlemen please. This is ridiculous. I really don't know what you are hoping to achieve."

"An overdraft," said Craney.

"Well I can assure you this is not the way to go about it," the bank manager replied somewhat indignantly.

"I went about it the normal way and you turned me down. I've been banking here for over five weeks." Craney sounded equally indignant.

"I'm afraid there's nothing I can do about it. It's totally out of my hands."

"So be it," I said slightly menacingly. "The CROUCHING community frowns upon your decision and will actively look to make your life as miserable as possible for as long as it takes for you to reverse your decision."

The bank manager's face reddened. "Is this some sort of threat?"

"I nodded, "yes it is a very serious threat. The CROUCHING community will now add you to its list of enemies alongside midgets, Chinese and certain Spar shops." With that I turned away from him and marched out of the bank, Craney clattering behind me.

The community was waiting outside and as I made my way back out onto the street a loud cheer rang out to greet me. It had been a good CROUCH, even Nikki and Gemma had turned up. I went over to greet them and Gemma gave me a big hug. "Fuck me mate, you really are making a name for yourself." At the same time Annie appeared and threw her arms around me.

"You did it Mr CROUCHER. It was brilliant." She was genuinely enthused.

"Girls, this is Annie. She's helping me organise the May Day CROUCH."

"I bet she is," laughed Nikki and then said to Annie, "you must have the patience of a saint."

Annie just smiled back and replied, "I'd do anything for Mr CROUCHER."

"Really?" Nikki looked at me and shook her head. She was about to say something when Craney grabbed her and dragged her away, Gemma following.

Jo joined us and prodded Annie. "Work time sweetie," she said and made a face that showed how much she was looking forward to it." Annie nodded and the girls gave me a kiss on either side of my face before rushing off.

As I watched them disappear, along with half a dozen fellow students, Nikki returned from Craney's grasp and said, "so much for you missing Lucy Mr Christie."

"I'll have you know they are valuable members of the CROUCHING community."

"I'm sure Lucy will be pleased as punch when you introduce her."

I grunted. "By the way am I still under surveillance?

"You sure are."

"So what now?" I asked.

"You can buy me a beer."

CHAPTER SEVENTEEN

PLOTTINGS PLANNINGS AND MISUNDERSTANDINGS

CROUCHING Community Membership 8,321

I made a few posts:

Sometimes we all have to make difficult decisions. Decisions that affect our very existence. Today whilst hiding in a bush it dawned on me that I had absolutely no idea where I was and no matter how loudly I barked nobody listened. Thus I made a life changing decision...never again will I eat Birds Eye potato waffles.

'The head of the CROUCHING community would like to offer an olive branch to all our yellow friends out there. If I am sent fifty photos from the Chinese community showing normal fanny positioning I will allow three Chinese people to attend the May Day CROUCH (in an observing role only - obviously). So get those legs open and cameras to hand; I'm velly velly excited.

I would like remind all community members to avoid the mobile 'topless' car wash service that continues to see innocent men having their wallets stolen whilst lost in a fog of soap suds and breasts. I had my wallet stolen on Tuesday, Friday and twice on Saturday.

In fridge related matters I have decided to open mine only on the quarter hours. By doing this I am able to calculate quite easily how many times I have opened it each day. So far I am averaging between ten and twelve times. Does this appear fairly standard?

The planned CROUCH outside the St Levan's Gate entrance of Devonport Dockyard has been postponed due to security issues. Yesterday the area was cordoned off after Devon and Cornwall police stopped a bus full of thalidomide sufferers. They accused them of bringing small arms into the country. The CROUCH will now be held later in the year.

In recent weeks there has been a welcome increase in the number of students attending CROUCHES. It was brought to my attention by one of them that I always bring each CROUCH to a close by reminding members to measure the size of their children's heads. As students in the main do not have children, they are not able to benefit from this piece of advice. I thought it would be nice if any of our members with more than one child would be prepared to allow these students to pop around to them once a month to measure one of the kids heads.

Due to the success of the recent midget hunt I have received numerous threats from our large headed foes, including one from a Serbian dwarf who has promised to fly to the U.K. and arrive mob handed with a bunch of machete wielding midgets to remove my knackers. With this in mind, I will in all future correspondence be using a photo of Craney.

This week's ham of the week is Waitrose honey crusted wafer thin. A slightly costlier choice but well worth treating your partner to on his or hers birthday etc.

Recent press reports have stated that I an unhinged. Whilst this may be true I wouldn't want people to allow this description of me to taint many worthwhile pursuits; such as leaning, climbing trees to a height of four feet, aggressive ham eating, hiding in bushes, kerb jumping and covering one's scrotum in Tippex.

The head of the CROUCHING community would like to remind all members that it is advisable to check under your bed EVERY time before turning off the lights.

During a recent on line discussion about sideways fannies it was mentioned that maybe I ought to pay for a Chinese hooker and this would settle the argument once and for all. So I bit the bullet and went on line and booked myself a fairly pricey Oriental escort only to find out that she had a penis. This has left me even more confused and with a severe case of hemorrhoids.

For all of you dead badger sniffers out there, of which I must admit I am one, I have just had a text message from a trusted source that there is a fairly decomposed black and white bastard just past the Lee Mill junction north bound on the A38.

It was with such tweets and posts that I amused myself as I waited for my phone to ring heralding Lucy's return. I must have checked it over fifty times by the time Gemma and the girls returned home from some day trip or other. "Kirk, she may not even get home until later tonight," she said trying to reassure me.

"I reckon she's already home. She's probably on her knees in front of her old man having a last nosh before her kids get home."

"Shut up you fucking idiot. That's not going to help is it?"

The conversation went back and forth as I came up with ever more ridiculous reasons as to why Lucy had yet to ring me. In the end she gave up; my demand of 'four pieces of fucking ham on a white fucking plate,' for my dinner was the last straw and she went to bed early leaving me pacing around with the big shoe on muttering at my phone to 'fucking ring you bastard.' Eventually I sat at the computer and hammered away; the interest that our Lloyd bank CROUCH had stirred was incredible. Indeed the number of views Lenny's video had got on You Tube was in the thousands. The community membership numbers were rocketing as we got more and more publicity and my inbox would have taken days to clear. Yet none of this mattered to me. All I wanted was to hear from Lucy and after a few hours I left the comfy chair for the cold kitchen floor. To make matters worse I woke face up, a sure sign that bad things were going to happen. I immediately reached for my phone and sure enough there was no message or missed call. I pulled myself up and flicked on the kettle; it was still dark but I didn't bother turning the light on. Instead I searched through my phone until I found Annie's number.

"Annie, I need you to get as many sheets as possible," I barked down the line as she answered with a sleepy hello.

"Mr CROUCHER," she said faintly. "What time is it?"

I couldn't see the time on my watch in the darkness but I took a guess anyway. "Ten past ten. Right, get a pen and some paper and make a list."

Annie groaned. "It's ten to five Mr CROUCHER. Are you mad?"

"Yes, you know I am, now get some paper will you," I responded impatiently. "Why do you need to ask that for?"

"Because it's ten to five."

I ignored her and went on, "we need sheets, lots of them. We'll hang them from every bridge in Plymouth advertising the CROUCH. You know, like they do with people's fortieth birthdays and stuff. You lot can hang them from your windows. Also we need spray paint. And lots of it. Get your art student lot to nick a load. And flags. Big ones..."

Annie finally managed to get a word in. "Why the hell can't this wait until later?"

"What?"

"This. All this list stuff. It can wait until later today. Are you pissed Mr CROUCHER?"

"No I haven't touched a drop. What day is it?"

I heard Annie sigh. "It's Saturday and very very early. I'll see you at the midday CROUCH and we can sort a list out then."

"Annie?"

"What?"

"Do you know anyone with a club foot?"

"Can I please go back to sleep you crazy man?"

"Sure, I'll see you later." I cut her off and went about trying to make a coffee in the darkness. I spilt hot water everywhere but eventually managed to fill my mug. I took it outside and stood sipping it listening to the morning chorus which at this time of year was truly beautiful. For some reason it again put the idea into my head as to whether I should start persecuting people with a wandering eye; you could never trust them that's for sure. Eventually, after what must have been almost an hour I went back inside the house feeling cold and depressed. The birds had stopped singing and another drizzly day was breaking. When Gemma came downstairs another hour later I was staring at myself in the hallway mirror.

"Have you been up all night again mate?"

I ignored the question and replied, "do I look alright to you Gem?"

"Yes you're beautiful," she said without looking at me. "How long have you been stood there for God's sake?"

"An hour or so. Do my eyes look alright?"

I heard an expletive come from the kitchen before I saw Gemma appear in the reflection. "Look mate, I know Lucy's due back any minute but fuck me, do you really have to spend so long in front of a mirror."

I ignored her and asked about me eyes again. "Do they look the same as normal?"

"Give it up Kirk will you. There's a coffee in the kitchen for you."

I did give it up, for about twenty minutes and then went straight back to the mirror. I even asked the girls to take a close look at me to see if I looked 'normal.' This went on for most of the morning until Gemma had obviously had enough and said she was going out. At least it appeared she didn't think I was likely to jump in front of a train anymore. As she slammed the front door behind her I shouted, "is it because I don't look right?"

An hour later I was out of the house myself and walking slowly to the final high noon CROUCH outside Mary Chang's takeaway. I should have been buzzing with anticipation but I was much too preoccupied with Lucy ringing and with stopping every fifty yards or so to look at myself in car wing mirrors. There was definitely a strange look in my eyes but I couldn't put my finger on it. For a few seconds I started to panic that I might be suffering from a wandering eye and had run to the nearest parked car to double check. I almost ran head first into a man walking a small dog, which started to bark hysterically at me. I apologised, mentioning the wandering eye situation but I'm not sure he quite understood what I was on about. I tried to calm myself by doing a spot of leaning on one of those wooden telegraph posts but it was all sticky with tar or something and I found myself cursing my leaning ambitions as a pointless piece of straight leg CROUCHING.

I spotted Annie as soon as Mary Chang's takeaway was in sight. She appeared to have pink and white hair now. As I got closer a few members saw me and a cheer went up. Someone, a student I guessed, was even carrying a flag with the CROUCHING man symbol on it and the words 'CROUCHING IN RANDOM PLACES' stencilled underneath. Once more the turnout was large, this time there must have been at least sixty or seventy students along with my usual regulars. There was no sign of Craney or big Andy, but Lenny was already filming away and I could hear Carter's trombone. I was treated to a hero's welcome and as much as I was worrying about my eyes I couldn't help but be somewhat self satisfied at the growth of the community. By the time I had greeted everyone there were easily more members than there was the day before. The pavement and the grass bank in front of the takeaway were absolutely packed with people ready to CROUCH. Annie came over a gave me a kiss then told me off about waking her up when she'd only got to bed at half past three. All I did was ask her if I looked normal.

I was beginning to worry that Mary Chang might not be in; normally by now she'd be screaming abuse out of the upstairs window of her flat. And that was when there had only been a handful of us CROUCHING. I noticed a couple of twitches at the curtain but nothing more than that. Regardless of this I had a job to do and when Lenny gave me the nod I raised an arm in the air and said loudly, "ladies and gentlemen, we are gathered here today for the last of our nigh noon CROUCHES, outside Mary Chang's Chinese Takeaway on Stone Barton Road, Plympton." I heard Carter shout 'sideways fanny' at the top of his lungs. "Today I will be performing a cheeky 150 degree double knee bend left foot heel lifted CROUCH. All animal noises and shouts of 'sideways fannies' are encouraged provided they are both loud and unseemly." With that I dropped into my CROUCH. It didn't take long for the first 'moos and barks' to start and within sixty seconds the noise was incredible. It took Mary Chang about thirty seconds longer before she appeared in the largest of the upstairs windows with an expression filled with pure rage. Her hair was bundled up in a towel, the reason I assumed that she had not appeared earlier.

"Oi you, fucking idiots. What you do here?" Mary had swung open the window and made her presence known thank God.

I raised a hand and waved up at her. "Good morning Mary. As you can see we are CROUCHING outside your fine establishment today. Isn't it splendid?"

"You! Fuck Christie!" Mary shouted at the top of her voice. A round of 'sideways fanny' shouts came back at her from the community. "Christie you fuck prick idiot. I fuck you up prick idiot."

"Now now Mary," I said calmly. "You ought to be thrilled that the CROUCHING community in all its glory has chosen to CROUCH outside your takeaway."

Mary of course was having none of it. "I fuck kill you Christie," she bellowed, even louder if that was possible. "I fuck kill you prick."

This was brilliant. Just what I had hoped for. "I would ask you to join us Mary," I shouted, "but unfortunately there is a ban in force currently on any form of Chinese participation."

For a moment I thought she might fall out the window. She leaned out as far as she possibly could and spat in my direction. "You scum prick. I kill you!" She was almost totally hysterical with anger now and the shouts of 'sideways fanny' just inflamed the stand off. She spat again then disappeared from view. I turned my attention back down to the takeaway below and wondered whether she might suddenly appear with a machete or something. However, her brief absence was quickly explained when she appeared back at the window with a bucket of water, which she emptied over the community members closest to the building. She managed to drench a good half dozen. A few seconds later a second bucket appeared but this time there was nobody in her range left to drench; that is except Craney who had arrived late without me noticing and had now taken up a position laying on his back directly under the window and was shouting, "drown me you yellow beauty," to much amusement.

Once Craney had received his desired wish I lifted an arm and shouted, "ladies and gentlemen of the CROUCHING community, thank you for attending our final high noon CROUCH outside Mary Chang's takeaway on Stone Barton Road or Seymour Road, they sort of meet here. Today, as you will have already noticed, we have been CROUCHING under a barrage of abuse, some of which you may find extremely distressing..." I didn't get any further due to the front door of the takeaway swinging open and Mary Chang bursting out waving what looked like some sort of ceremonial sword above her head.

"I kill you Christie prick idiot," she shouted at me her eyes blazing with anger.

For a moment I stood smiling at her as she made her way towards me through the rapidly parting community. Then I shouted, "It's the Boxer uprising!" And turned to run. She was never going to catch me in a million years and I had plenty of time to slow down, turn and shout various offensive remarks such as, "give us back our opium," and "Hong Kong Phooey was a nonce." Eventually she gave up and I stopped running to turn and face her about fifty yards up the road. She was waving the sword around like Errol Flynn on speed and shouting stuff about me being a 'fuck idiot pig fuck.' I watched her stomp back to the takeaway still shouting abuse at everyone and half heartedly waving the sword. Craney shouted "what size are your feet?" which caused Mary to scream a final round of obscenities before going back inside the takeaway and slamming the door shut behind her.

When everything had calmed down I made a further announcement to the stunned community many of whom were looking shell shocked. "I apologise for all the unnecessary commotion today; I believe it to be a side affect of sideways fanny syndrome. This is the final of our high noon CROUCHES and indeed the last CROUCH until next Sunday's May Day CROUCH. I look forward to seeing you all there for what will no doubt be a landmark in CROUCHING history. For now we will do a second, short, thirty second CROUCH and don't forget to measure your children's heads at least once a week." There was a big shout of 'water melons' from the general direction of Carter.

I quickly did the rounds apologising to people for the interruption of the CROUCH and then rounded up big Andy and the lads for a meeting at the Josh to discuss the May Day CROUCH. I was checking my phone yet again as Annie and Jo appeared next to me. I looked up smiling and said, "can you come up the pub now? We are going to sort out the May Day CROUCH."

"We are honoured," said Jo smiling broadly and Annie gave me a kiss on the cheek and asked if a few of their friends could come too. I agreed and left them too it, grabbing Craney who was absolutely dripping wet and made my way to big Andy's transit van.

"Do you think your student mate fucks for cash?" Carter asked as we headed to the pub.

I turned to look over my shoulder. "Who Annie?"

"The tall punk one. Is that her name is it?"

"Yeah, Annie. I don't know mate," I answered honestly. "Probably. All students do these days don't they?"

Big Andy joined in the conversation. "I'd fucking give her one that's for sure. And her little pal with the massive tits."

"Yeah but you have to think about the Chlamydia problem," I said.

Carter seemed to agree with me and said, "true mate. Find out how much she charges for a blow job." And so the conversation went until we pulled up outside the pub. It was the longest I had been in two days without checking my phone.

The bar was already full of community members; the landlord owed me a good few drinks for the amount of custom I was bringing in these days. I immediately peered at myself in the optics mirror and decided that there was definitely something not quite right with me. Someone handed me a bottle of Pils and a ten minutes later I was sat at a corner table surrounded by the CROUCHING community's finest, preparing to organise the defining moment in the brief history of my obsession with the bending of knees. Annie and Jo and a couple of young male students had joined me, Craney, big Andy, Lenny, Carter, Dan and Stan squeezed around the small table and for the next half hour we hammered out a plan of action covering everything from bombarding the press to spraying most of Plympton in CROUCHING graffiti. I continually hammered home that we were the centre of the CROUCHING world and had to ensure what we did surpassed everywhere else, especially Molly's lot in New York. Annie proved her worth by offering huge support from the local students as well as students from many other universities across the country. When everything was agreed on Carter immediately began nudging me and gesturing towards Annie as the rest of the gathering headed back to the bar.

"Have you ever blown a trombone?" I asked her hoping she'd catch my drift.

"You mean like your mate's one?"

"Yeah *just* like that," I said trying to sound serious.

"Cheeky bugger. What kind of girl do you take me for?" She had a wonderfully cheeky expression on her face. "To be honest I'm more of a double bass sort of chick."

I laughed and made a shrugging gesture at Carter who shook his head and headed over to the pool table. Turning back to Annie I asked, "do I look alright today?"

"In what sense?"

"Just sort of not normal."

Annie laughed and said, "you're never normal Mr CROUCHER. That's why we all love you. Talking of which, have you heard from your lady yet?"

I shook my head. "Not a thing."

"Poor old Mr CROUCHER," she said pouting and put her arms around me. Looking over her shoulder I could see Carter frowning at me and big Andy making obscene gestures. I mouthed 'fuck off' at them and pulled away from Annie's embrace. "Are you sure you are okay doing all this stuff for us?"

"I can't wait to get started," she replied enthusiastically and I believed her. I was about to ask her to look at my eyes when Carter let out a huge roar of "gatage!"

I looked across to the pool table to see him waving his cue and Dan who was shouting back, "fuck off that's no way gatage!"

"What on earth are they on about? Asked Annie.

"Oh it's a game we play on the pool table involving the fire grate placed across the middle as you can see."

"Yeah but that would be gratage surely?"

I looked at her and shook my head as if she was simple. "We used to play 'shit pool' until the landlord banned it. You'd cover all but one of the balls in chocolate and the other remaining one in shit. A load of you would take in turns potting the balls until there was just one left and whoever's turn it was had to put this ball in their mouth."

Annie made a noise of disgust. "That's awful."

"It was better than 'string pool' I can tell you."

"Really? Do I want to know?"

I smiled and said, "put it this way, only men could play it and it involved a lot of running

around the table keeping your eyes fixed on a particular string. A very particular string."
Before Annie could comment another roar of 'gatage!' swept across the bar. I could see Jo
looking a little concerned as were the rest of the students. Annie didn't appear to be in the
least bothered until a pool ball came flying past us and a few minutes later gave me a kiss
and left. I stayed for a couple more hours, mainly because Nikki and Gemma turned up
making the most of a day with no kids. The game of 'gate pool' ended in acrimony after big
Andy snapped Dan's cue in half and threatened to shove it up his arse. Shortly after which
Craney, who was still wet, grabbed me and demanded that we carry out a pre May Day
CROUCH arson campaign, which, as much as it appealed to me I had to make him settle on
a night of graffiti fun with big Andy's newly 'acquired' yellow, city council, road marking
spray. Before I left for home I demanded that Gemma ring Lucy's mobile, which she finally
did when I bought her a double vodka and surprise surprise it went to voicemail. She left a
message saying that she hoped she had had a good holiday and to get in touch.

"Did it ring for a while or go straight to answer phone?" I demanded even before Gemma
had ended the call properly.

"It went straight to answer phone mate," she replied and grabbed the vodka from me.

I wasn't sure if this was a good thing or not and I left the noisy pub feeling agitated. It
took me ages to get home as I kept stopping every couple of minutes to look at myself in
car wing mirrors. I couldn't put my finger on it but something was definitely not quite right.
When I finally got home I immediately went to the computer and had a look on Lucy's
Facebook page to see if there was any activity; there wasn't. I sent a message asking her
where the hell she was and then began going through all the e mails and messages that were
now getting out of hand. I would need to sit here for days to answer every one. I did smile
when I read one from the manager of Comet who was complaining about our recent
CROUCH outside the store. I immediately made the following post on the CROUCHING
In Random Places website:

I received an abusive e mail today from the manager of Comet, Marsh Mills in relation to our recent CROUCH outside the premises. He has threatened to sell all of us a load of extended warranties should we ever CROUCH there again.

Kirkland Christie   Head of the CROUCHING Community

I chuckled to myself as I shut the computer down and went back to the mirror in the hallway. I was still there shouting 'cunt!' at my reflection over and over when a drunk Gemma fell in through the front door and joined in with me. She was just getting fed up with it and no doubt about to tell me to 'shut the fuck up' when I heard big Andy's horn beeping. I gave a last shout, kissed Gemma who looked like she was about throw up, grabbed a jacket and went out into the dark night. Craney looked like he was about to carry out some sort of SAS exercise; a balaclava and black jumper giving him an even more worrying look than he normally had. To top it off a long spliff jutted out from a home made hole which looked closer to where his nose should be than his mouth.

"Hello matey," he said full of excitement. I'm all ready for any places which have

CCTV coverage."

"Top man Mr Crane," I said meaning it. I could always rely on him to go the extra mile for the CROUCHING cause.

Our first stop was St Mary's roundabout which was the coming together of Plympton's three main trunk roads and as such was always busy. It took a good ten minute wait until all three roads were empty. Craney then ran onto the mini roundabout and sprayed a large yellow stick man CROUCHING with the legend, 'CROUCHING IN RANDOM PLACES' below it. I had to admit Craney had done a first class job and it gave us the start we needed to crack on with the task in hand.

For the next three hours each one of us had come close to being run over by a taxi as we went about spraying as many roads as possible. Craney wanted to spray St Mary's church but I managed to dissuade him. Instead he settled on the local Co-op and Lloyds bank. We finished with a couple of verges under a flyover on the A38 before I risked life and limb running out into the darkness on the dual carriageway and spraying a huge CROUCHING man and ten feet high letters proclaiming, 'THE CROUCHING COMMUNITY IS HERE FOR ALL (EXCEPT THE CHINESE).'

I asked big Andy to drop me off at Hall Graves and Lee; I felt in need of a late night solo CROUCH at the spiritual home of the CROUCHING Community. Craney was desperate to join me but I insisted I wanted to be alone. I climbed up onto the low wall as I had done dozens of time before and slipped into a nice and easy 140 degree double knee bend CROUCH. For the first time in what felt like weeks the clouds lifted and I was able to think clearly. I considered breaking into Lucy's house. It seemed the logical choice and I wondered why I hadn't thought of it up until now. I made the ten minute walk to Lucy's house, struggling in the dark to pick it out; I had only been past it once before. When I got there it was obviously occupied, the curtains were drawn and two cars were in the drive, one of which was Lucy's. I could make out the light from a TV screen in the bedroom. I considered going around the back but in the end felt so depressed at the whole thing I just lifted off one of the driveway gates and walked slowly home. When I reached Gemma's I threw it into the front garden next to the traffic light, went inside and stared at myself in the hallway mirror once more. I was still standing there when Gemma came downstairs hours later.

"The kitchen floor not good enough for you any more? She sort of growled, obviously suffering from a hangover.

"Have you heard back from Lucy?" I asked, ignoring her sarcasm.

"Nothing mate. Coffee?"

I followed her into the kitchen and told her what I had seen a few hours before.

"Well in that case I'm sure she'll be in touch today. How did the spraying go?"

I gave her a brief run down before grabbing the coffee and going back to the mirror. Just to round off my morning the ex wife rang to tell me what an embarrassment I was and that she was changing her shifts so that I wouldn't have to look after Zak anymore. He didn't want to see me for the time being she went on and her father was going to have the sausage kings for the next few weeks. It was just the sort of kick in the balls I needed and I threw my phone on the floor and began shouting "cunt!" in earnest at myself in the mirror.

Gemma shouted at me to shut up, then when I told her what the ex wife's call had been about all she said was, "I told you so you knob."

I gave up with the mirror and went and lay face down on the kitchen floor. "It's all going wrong Gem. Everything's falling apart," then added, "fucking midgets."

"She'll be in touch mate," Gem said lying on the floor next to me, more from the hangover than an act of solidarity. "And so will your son. He's probably embarrassed at having his dad plastered all over the papers and on the box." Ten minutes later she had rolled over onto her back and was fast asleep.

I decided to ring Lucy; now I knew she was home all bets were off. The call went straight to voicemail. "Where the fuck are you fat head? Ring me immediately." My tone wasn't particularly loving but I wasn't in the best of moods. I left Gemma snoring and went back to the mirror and spent an hour shouting 'cunt' at myself. I stopped to let the girls in when Gemma's sister dropped them off shortly before midday and they took no time in getting a couple of chairs so they could join me with my shouting. Gemma finally pulled herself off the kitchen floor and screamed "enough!" The girls shot upstairs and I headed for the computer.

Our night of 'yellow' vandalism had already created a huge buzz online and there were loads of photos being uploaded. I stared blankly at the screen not really taking it all in. My mind was elsewhere. In the end, after another run in with Gemma I walked to Nikki's to try and find some sympathy. However she was out and I ended up climbing on her shed roof and CROUCHING, only to fall into her neighbour's garden causing another row. I told the neighbour that I was the head of the CROUCHING community and had every right to fall into his garden as it was a CROUCHING related incident. He told me in no uncertain terms to get off his property immediately and after I called him a 'Tory midget sympathiser' I stomped off back to Gemma's only stopping to ring Lucy again and demand she rang me back. She didn't.

CHAPTER EIGHTEEN

ANNIE I'M NOT YOUR DADDY

CROUCHING Community Membership 9,003

Whilst I had been shouting 'cunt!' at myself for hours Annie and her student pals had been busily painting sheets which were to be hung from every road, rail and foot bridge in the city. Each one had a CROUCHING stick man on it with the words 'MAY DAY CROUCH SUNDAY 1ST MAY AT HIGH NOON OUTSIDE DEVON PINE FURNITURE SHOP EXETER STREET PLYMOUTH'. I had been worried that there was too much information to take in but when Annie arrived to pick me up in her little Fiat I was thrilled with the results. It was close to midnight and I had been fretting for hours about Lucy, so spending the night with Annie racing around the A38 was a good diversion. It had been agreed that Annie's crowd would be responsible for all the banners and flags etc and it was my good fortune to be chaperoned by her for the night. I climbed into the passenger seat and lost sight of my feet amongst the empty cans of drink and chocolate wrappers.

"Hey Mr CROUCHER," Annie said breezily and lent over and kissed me.

"Hi sweetheart. This car's a shit pit."

She laughed, throwing her head backwards. "I'm a student, shut your mouth. And anyway, I've been painting sheets for the last twenty four hours or the car would have been gleaming seeing as I am chauffeuring such an important man."

It was my turn to laugh. "And don't you fucking forget it."

"Did you bring the big shoe?"

I shook my head and answered, "sorry sweetheart, not tonight."

She made a face and started the car, pulling quickly away before asking, "where first then sir?"

I thought for a moment then replied, "do I look funny to you?"

"What?"

"Do I look funny? You know, sort of different?"

"You look beautiful as always."

I shook my head and pulled down the sun visor but there was no mirror. "Fucking Italians," I muttered in reference to the Fiat.

"Where are we going Mr CROUCHER?" Annie asked again.

"The Plympton flyover. Deep Lane it's called or something. Anyway just go up the A38 and I'll tell you where to turn off."

Annie talked incessantly as we made our way to our first destination. She told me about how many students would be out across Plymouth tonight and how many she hoped to get to the May Day CROUCH itself. I sat and said nothing; happy for her to prattle on to herself. My mind was elsewhere. It took us less than ten minutes to get to the flyover and I gestured to Annie to go over the bridge and park the car up a quiet lane just beyond the junction.

"I knew it," exclaimed Annie. "You dirty old man"

I turned and grinned at her in the darkness. "The head of the CROUCHING community's days of car intimacy are long past."

"Car intimacy?" Annie burst out laughing.

I ignored her and got out of the car and took a deep breath of the fresh nighttime air. Annie walked around to me and came close enough that I could smell her faint perfume. "You're so different Mr CROUCHER. You are a very special man."

"I'm a cunt," I said and walked past her to the boot.

"Well your full of fun tonight Mr CROUCHER. I take it you still haven't seen Lucy?"

"No," was all I said and opened the boot. There was a neat pile of folded sheets inside and a couple of boxes of plastic cable ties. Very organised. I reached in and pulled out a sheet. Annie grabbed an end and between us we pulled it fully open. "I'm impressed," I said honestly. "Are they all like this?" Annie nodded. They were about 100 times better than anything I could have come up with. The black lettering was bold and neat; the CROUCHING man perfectly balanced. "I fucking love it," I said smiling at Annie.

"You better do. Hours of my life that I'll never get back went into those."

"Right," I said, finally getting into the task at hand. "Grab some of those cable ties. We'll put one up on each side of the bridge."

It took us almost half an hour before I was satisfied. Annie ignored my constant cursing, instead poking fun at me for my foul mood. However, when the job was done I smiled at her, knowing how good the banners looked. Annie gave me a high five, which I somewhat reluctantly accepted and we headed back to the car.

"Where next Mr CROUCHER?" Annie asked as I fastened my seat belt.

"We'll do three more bridges up as far as Ivybridge or so and then I'll buy you a coffee at the Little Chef."

"And pancakes?" Annie clapped her hands like a child, reminding me of the seventeen year age difference between us. I nodded and she hastily reversed back onto the road and made for the A38 and our next bridge. I spent almost the entire journey craning my neck to try and look into wing mirror much to Annie's amusement.

"Mr CROUCHER, you look fine. Honestly."

"Well, I don't feel fine," I mumbled and spent the next couple of hours trying to appear keen whilst at the same time asking Annie if I looked alright. She showed unlimited patience with me and did all she could to lift my spirits and keep my mind from drifting to Lucy, but by the time we were sat in the Little Chef she could no longer hold back.

"Come on Mr CROUCHER. We've done brilliantly tonight and I've had loads of texts from all the rest of the gang. Plymouth is awash with CROUCHING banners." She showed me her phone. "Look, even the station has been done."

I smiled somewhat sadly at her and said, "It's brilliant Annie. Everything you and your student mob are doing for the community is superb. I truly am in your debt."

"Don't be ridiculous, I've loved every minute of it." I knew she was telling the truth. She went on, "It's Lucy isn't it?"

I nodded. "She just doesn't want to get in touch. I am lost without her." I meant it. I felt empty.

"I don't have any answers Mr CROUCHER. But I will help you in anyway I can. I mean it."

"Thanks Annie, but there's nothing anyone can do. It's down to her."

Still holding my hand she said, "well you have me now and I'm going to make sure you are okay Mr CROUCHER. I won't let you get depressed."

I smiled at her. "If only it was that simple Annie."

We sat drinking coffee for over an hour; I listened to Annie as she kept me abreast of all the night's efforts by her friends, which were impressive and about her love of movies and the punk culture. I nodded where necessary and added the odd comment but for the best part let her do all the talking. I was glad of the distraction to be honest. When we finally got up to go I felt a little better and immediately walked to the first car I saw and looked in the wing mirror.

"Are you sure I look okay?"

Annie swore at me and dragged me away. Twenty minutes later we were stood on the large flyover high above Marsh Mills roundabout, by far the busiest intersection on Plymouth's roads. In all we hung up five sheets; it took ages as the wind had whipped up and just as we were about to tie the sixth and last one the sky opened and a huge burst of rain began to fall. We both cursed and ran for the car which was parked in a lay by about 200 yards up the road. By the time we reached it we were both soaked, although Annie had the benefit of having the final sheet wrapped around her.

"Fucking hell," I gasped slamming the door behind me. Annie was laughing and after I while I joined her and we sat, drenched, giggling like children.

"What about this last sheet?" She asked me, throwing it onto the back seat.

A sudden thought came into my head and once it had I knew I had no way of ignoring it. "We'll place it on Lucy's front lawn," I announced.

"Are you sure?" Annie asked as she started the engine at the second attempt. "No, of course you're sure. Tell me how to get there."

I guided Annie through the empty streets; the rain easing to a steady downpour and considered what a good idea it was. Lucy would see the sheet when she pulled back her bedroom curtains and know I was thinking of her. She was bound to call me.

"Slow down a bit," I said and gestured to Annie to pull over to the kerb. "I think it's that one," I pointed at the dark houses.

We got out, Annie carrying the flag and walked the few yards to Lucy's house, which was now easy to pick out due to its missing driveway gate. "I took it to Gemma's," I said gesturing at the gatepost. I didn't turn to look to see if Annie knew what I was on about. I was too busy deciding where to place the sheet.

"Give the sheet to me," I said quietly to Annie. I turned to her but she shook her head and whispered, "one end each. Where do you want to put it?"

Between us we laid the sheet as perfectly as was possible; I grabbed a couple of large stones from the rockery of sorts in the corner of the garden. All in all it was the ultimate calling card from the head of the CROUCHING community to his most cherished. I got back in the car and let out a sigh of relief at a good night's work completed. Then I grabbed the rear view mirror and shouted 'cunt!' at myself half a dozen times much to

Annie's delight. When she pulled up outside Gemma's it was gone four in the morning.

"I would ask you in Annie but to be honest I expect I'll be shouting 'cunt' at myself in the mirror for the rest of the night and I wouldn't want you to have to face an angry Gemma."

Annie leant forward and kissed me on the lips. It was about as delicate a kiss as you could possibly imagine. "It's okay Mr CROUCHER, I understand. It's been a fun night."

"Say a big thank you to all the others from me," I said meaning it.

She drove off into the night leaving me stood motionless in the rain. I didn't move until long after the sound of the little Fiat had faded and only then when a small tortoiseshell cat rubbed up against my legs. I reached down to stroke it and made my way to the front door. I looked across at Lucy's gate resting haphazardly in the front garden and wondered whether she realised it had been me who took it. No doubt she would put two and two together when she woke up to the banner glaring up at her. Saying that she probably put two and two together as soon as she saw the gate was missing; I mean, who else is going to randomly pinch a garden gate?

The house was deathly quiet as I entered and this suited me fine. I had spent all night listening to Annie chatter away and the peace was welcome. I stripped off completely naked, throwing my clothes in the washing machine and made a coffee. As I sipped it I considered ringing Lucy. I was sure I had her home number written down somewhere. In the end I just stood and drank my coffee and dwelt on whether a night face down on the kitchen floor naked would help my mood. Eventually I went to the hallway mirror to stare at myself and was still standing there when the girls came down sometime a few hours later. They were most impressed that I was naked and even joined in with a bout of 'cunt' shouting which I couldn't help starting when they had pointed at my nether regions. To say Gemma was unimpressed when she came down twenty minutes later was a slight understatement and when the girls asked if they too could strip naked she politely informed me that I may be causing a problem.

"Kirk, what the fucking hell are you doing now?" She roared. "For fuck's sake this is getting out of hand. Where the fuck are your clothes?"

I didn't even turn to look at her such was my focus on the face in the mirror. I continued to shout 'cunt' over and over until Gemma eventually dragged me away. "Do I look strange to you Gemma?" I asked completely oblivious of the unfolding drama.

"Get me a towel off the banister girls, quickly." I heard Gemma say and a minute later she was wrapping the large fluffy, ever so slightly damp towel around me and pushing me into the kitchen. I heard her shoe the girls into the lounge and felt her arms around my waist holding me tightly. "What the hell's going on Kirk? Are you with me?"

I nodded, said I was fine and asked if she had a mirror to hand.

CHAPTER NINETEEN

THE ARRIVAL OF DICK VAN DYKE

CROUCHING Community Membership 9211

I left another voicemail demanding Lucy ring me straight away and spent a few hours laying face down on the kitchen floor. The girls walked around me not taking a blind bit of notice to my unusual relaxing position. They asked if they could walk around the lounge with the big shoe on. At least someone understood the benefit of starting the day like this I thought. Gemma came in the back door carrying an empty washing bin and asked if I intended staying on the floor all day and where the fuck had the gate come from.

"It's Lucy's," I said not bothering to lift my head.

"Well that's hardly going to help is it? By the way your phone's been driving me mad." She tossed it down to me. There were loads of messages from friends and community members congratulating me on the banner campaign. The call I had been waiting for finally came at some point in the afternoon. I was still on the kitchen floor.

"You're alive then?" I said answering the phone, immediately regretting my sarcastic tone.

"Kirk, what the fuck?" Lucy's voice was full of anger.

"What?" I said and waited.

"Don't you dare," Lucy snapped. "Don't you dare give me what. You know exactly fucking well what."

"The gate?" I asked casually.

"Was that you as well? I should have guessed."

"You mean there are potentially other gate collectors out there?"

"For fuck's sake Kirk. Why put that fucking flag in the garden? You're such a twat?" I could tell that for once the term 'twat' was not one of endearment.

"Says the woman who is apparently in love with me but can't be arsed to even send me a text."

"I'm not doing this Kirk. I am not fucking doing this." The phone line went dead.

"Fuck!" I shouted and threw my phone across the kitchen.

"That went well then," said Gemma appearing in the doorway.

I banged my head repeatedly on the kitchen floor until Gemma grabbed hold of me. "You need to calm down mate," she said as I got up rubbing my head.

"I need some fresh air. I need to think."

I went to find a pair of shoes but couldn't make it past the hallway mirror. What I saw bore little resemblance to how I saw myself. "Cunt!" I started shouting again until Gemma once more pulled me away. She found me a pair of trainers and pushed me out of the front door telling me to "calm the fuck down."

I found myself heading towards the ex wife's place which was only going to go one way but I was incapable of changing direction. I knocked on her door loudly and was greeting by an angry looking ex wife asking tersely what I wanted.

"To see my son," I answered truthfully.

"He's at school Kirk. You know, back to school? Christ you look like you haven't seen a bed in a week; have you looked at yourself lately?"

"You'd be surprised," I answered flatly.

"Christ you are an embarrassment."

"Actually I'm the head of the CROUCHING community," I said proudly.

"You're pathetic," she snapped. "Listen to you. It's no wonder your son wants nothing to do with you. Can you imagine what it's like for him seeing his father splattered across the newspapers and on the TV?"

"I thought he'd be very proud."

"For chasing midgets?"

"I wasn't chasing them, I was hunting them."

The ex wife let out a sound of exasperation. "For God's sake Kirk. Listen to yourself."

I ignored her. "When can I see my son?"

She slammed the door in my face leaving me standing on the doorstep. I opened the letter box and shouted, "I'm the head of the CROUCHING community!" With that I turned abruptly and noticed a neighbour who had stopped cleaning his car to stare at me. I walked towards him and shouted full blast, "I'm Dick Van fucking Dyke!" I've no idea where that came from but the bloke quickly headed back to his house leaving his car covered in soap suds. I considered finishing cleaning it but knew I had an appointment at Lucy's house that was becoming more and more urgent as each minute passed. On the way I stopped outside the Colebrook fish and chips shop for a short CROUCH, which involved a lot of barking much to the owner's wrath. It did amuse the queuing customers though and helped released a bit of my ever building tension. When I reached Lucy's house I immediately saw the banner had been removed but Lucy's car was still parked on the drive. I walked purposefully up to the front door and rang the bell. After what felt like an hour wait the door finally swung open and a woman of similar age to my mother appeared. She looked at me suspiciously; peering over the top of her half rim spectacles.

"Yes?" She said slowly and deliberately, dragging out the word.

"I'm here to see Lucy," I replied, trying to sound like I was expected.

"I'm afraid she's still in hospital." Alarms bells began to ring in my head. "Are you a friend?" The woman who I guessed was Lucy's mother gave me a suspicious look.

"I'm the head of the CROUCHING community," I stated firmly, causing the woman to remove her spectacles and frown.

"I see," she said coldly. "Am I to presume it was your handiwork that I woke up to this morning?" She gestured towards the garden.

I nodded vigorously then said, "is she going to be alright? You see I'm in love with her. In fact we are both very much in love with each other."

The woman took a step back and closed the door slightly. "I don't know who the hell you are or what you are going on about for that matter but I suggest you leave this minute."

I ignored her demand and asked, "is she in Derriford hospital?"

"Yes but..."

I cut her off before she could finish. "Right, I'll go and visit her." With that I turned and marched out of the drive shouting over my shoulder that I knew where she could get a new gate. I heard her shouting something at me but I was on a mission. I had to see Lucy. I marched to the nearest taxi rank which took me twenty minutes, my mind doing somersaults at the news that Lucy was in hospital. I kept saying 'shit' over and over as it dawned on me that I may just have made the worst mistake of my life. On top of this I found myself panicking with regard to whether Lucy would die. No, she had rang me and she sounded okay.

 As the taxi approached the main entrance of the huge building I found myself looking at the large scar across my forearm, the reason for my most recent visit to A & E. Twelve months ago I had decided it was a good idea to chop my arm off with a samurai sword which had been hanging from a wall at a friend's house. Sixteen stitches and a week in the nutty farm had been the result. I was still thinking about this when I paid the taxi driver and headed into the hospital reception. I waited twenty minutes before being told what ward Lucy was on. It took another twenty minutes to reach it.

 "I've come to see Lucy Reynolds," I said loudly to one of the three nurses gathered at the ward entrance.

 "Ah Lucy," she said smiling. "Yes she's just down there on the left." She pointed down the corridor and added, "third door."

 "How's she doing?" I asked, unsure if I wanted to know.

 "Really well," the nurse replied and went back to her business.

 When I reached Lucy's room I stopped and peered through the window. I could feel my heart trying to burst through my chest. And there she was, sitting up in the bed reading a magazine. Her skin had an ever so slight tan and even without a hint of make up or the customary lipstick, she looked wonderful. I stood staring at her through the window for a minute; watching as she reached for a glass of water. The room was full of flowers and cards, more than enough evidence to suggest she had been here for a good few days. All my longing for her flooded through my body and once again I knew she was the one; the shining beacon in my dark world. Eventually I took a deep breath, opened the door and walked in. She immediately looked up from her magazine no doubt expecting to see a nurse or doctor. When she saw it was me her expression went from at first astonishment to then one of horror.

"Kirk, you can't be here." She managed to blurt out.

"I had to see you."

"My husband's on his way for Christ's sake."

"So?" I shrugged. "I don't care."

"Well I do Kirk. You have to leave."

"You sound like your mum," I said smiling at her.

"What?" The expression of horror returned.

"I guess it was your mother. I called round your house. How do you think I found out you were in here?"

"You went to my house?" Her mouth fell open.

"Yeah," I grinned.

"Kirk, for fuck's sake!" Lucy snapped, glaring at me.

"She didn't even seem impressed when I told her I was the head of the CROUCHING community."

"Oh my God, what have you done Kirk? Why?"

"I told her that I love you. Actually I think I told her we are in love."

Lucy put her head in her hands and let out a low moan, then muttered, "Jesus," over and over.

I walked over to her side and asked, "do I look normal by the way?" Ignoring her obvious discomfort.

She lifted her head out of her hands and replied, "you look like shit. I hardly recognised you."

"I've not been very well," I offered by way of explanation.

Lucy let out a gasp and snapped, "You've not been very well? I'm hardly having a picnic am I? And now all this extra crap. You're such a fucking idiot."

I started at the love of my life refusing to listen to the words she was showering me with. "I love you fat head," I said quietly.

"Get out Kirk. Go." Lucy pointed at the door. "God knows what damage you've done." She flung her head back into her pillows saying, "fuck, fuck ,fuck." Then when seeing that I hadn't moved shouted, "get out!"

A nurse appeared in the doorway, obviously hearing Lucy shouting. I looked at her and said, "I love her" which led Lucy to respond with "get him out of here." The nurse escorted me out of the ward and pointed me in the direction of the elevators. On entering the first that arrived I made no attempt to ignore my reflection in the mirrored walls. "Cunt!" I shouted at myself. "You're a cunt!" The three other people in the lift said nothing, not that I would have noticed anyway. Maybe they thought I had lost a loved one. Maybe I just had.

When I reached the fresh air I took three large gulps to calm myself, walked across the road and slumped down on the nearest bench next to a rather fat woman wearing a dressing gown. I turned to look at her and saw she was rolling a cigarette. "Smoking kills," I said shaking my head.

"What are you, a doctor?" The fat woman said putting the roll up in her mouth.

I shook my head. "No. I am the head of the CROUCHING community."

The woman frowned, lit the roll up and took a long drag. "The what?"

"It doesn't matter," I said softly and closed my eyes. I sat for a long time; the sun warming my cheeks. I sat there until my phone buzzed in my pocket. "Hello yes?" I answered on auto pilot.

"Hello Mr CROUCHER," purred Annie. "What you up to?"

"I'm sunbathing outside Derriford hospital."

"Why?" There was a hint of concern in Annie's voice.

"It's a Chlamydia scare," I said to her amusement, then added, "I need you to come and get me."

"Has something happened?"

"I'll explain later. Can you pick me up?"

"You'll have to give me an hour. I'm still at Uni."

"Okay, I'll be sat on a bench with my eyes closed outside the main entrance." I cut her off before she could reply.

Ten minutes later my phone buzzed again. This time it was a text. Not just a text. It was from Lucy. It took me almost five minutes before I could bring myself to open it. When I did I wished I hadn't. It said: 'Kirk you have ruined everything. Do NOT turn up here or at my house ever again. I MEAN IT.' I was still staring at it three quarters of an hour later when Annie arrived. I nodded at her and ambled over to the car ignoring the queue growing behind her. I got in and immediately noticed how pink her jumper was; it was very pink and very fluffy. Annie saw me looking at it and said, "it's great isn't it? I picked it up for a quid in Oxfam."

"It's very pink," was all I could offer.

Annie pulled away and as soon as we were on the main road she turned and asked, "okay Mr CROUCHER, what's happened? And don't say nothing because I can see something's not right."

I let out a sigh and told her everything.

"You do realise her husband's going to kill you," was the first thing Annie said when I had finished my sorry tale of woe.

I shrugged. "I'm way past worrying about things like that." I was about to add something but instead just grabbed the rear view mirror and started the 'cunt' shouting once more. Eventually, when she had the opportunity, Annie pulled over into a bus bay and turned to me saying, "calm down Mr CROUCHER. It's going to be okay." She reached over and stroked my face in an attempt to calm me. Once she was satisfied I was back with her she said, "come on, lets get you home," and for the rest of the journey I remained quiet. When we arrived at Gemma's I went straight to the mirror but Annie dragged me away and into the kitchen.

"Where's the big shoe?" I said, looking around the kitchen.

"I'll find it," Annie said and disappeared. When she returned a few minutes later I was already laying in my customary position. She placed the big shoe down on the lino next to me and then laid on top of me. "I'm not moving until you're okay," she said into my ear.

"You're fucking heavy woman," I moaned.

"Tough."

I had no idea how long we laid there. I enjoyed the feeling of Annie's weight on me. It gave me a strange sense of security. Every now and again she would whisper something in my ear but I paid no heed to what was being said. My mind was too full of varying emotions. Eventually I must have drifted off to sleep because the next thing I recalled was hearing Nikki's voice and the smell of cigarette smoke.

"Ah sleeping beauty has woken," I heard Gemma say.

I rolled stiffly over onto my back; Annie was nowhere to be seen. "What day is it?" I asked Gemma as I pulled myself up. She was stood by the back door with Nikki, smoking.

Shaking her head she said to her, "I swear I'm going to buy him those fucking Y fronts with each day of the week on the front."

"What day is it?" I said again.

"It's Monday Kirk," said Nikki laughing. She pointed to the clock on the cooker. "And it's ten past ten!"

I looked at my watch and was glad to see it was working again. "Where's Annie?" I asked as I poured a glass of water.

"I sent her home when I got back," said Gemma. "Well about half an hour after I got back. I poured her a large glass of wine first. Poor girl deserves a medal. She was all for staying here until you woke up but I thought you might end up sleeping all night. And before you say it, she told me all about Lucy. What the fuck got into that head of yours?" She raised a hand and added, "no don't answer that."

"Have you heard from her?"

"No mate and if I were you I'd leave her be for a while."

"Was Annie okay?"

Gemma grabbed a wine glass from the draining board and filled it with some of her cheap white stuff. "She's a sweetie. I couldn't believe it when I came in to see her lying on top of you. The girls thought it was brilliant. She said she'll ring you in the morning."

"It's been a very bad day," I said and told them about my visit to the ex wife's. Both the women shook their heads at me and their looks told me all I needed to know. I left the wine and grabbed a beer from the fridge along with a few slices of ham. My brain was so addled I couldn't even tell if it was regular or wafer thin. I left the girls to their smoking and made my way to the computer. The one benefit from collapsing on the kitchen floor was that I know felt fully refreshed. I spent the night split between hammering away on the computer and staring into the hallway mirror. The website was awash with various plans for May Day

CROUCHES around the world and there were literally hundreds of photos of banners and flags advertising the event. It took me hours just to go through my e-mails and messages. I needed a P.A. When I had finally answered as many questions and queries as I could I made a tweet about something that had been bugging me:

Recently I have become concerned that I may be turning into Dick Van Dyke. Is this a symptom of Chlamydia? I was hoping it might be a ham related side affect.

I then spent a good half hour staring at photos of Lucy on her Facebook page. I still refused to accept I had done anything wrong. I thought she loved me. Surely she would want me to find her whilst she was in hospital. However, this *didn't* seem to be the case when she rang me just after Gemma had left to take the kids to school.

"Hello yes?"

"What got into you Kirk?" Lucy said without preamble.

"I don't follow."

I heard her sigh. "Don't start Kirk. What on earth made you go to my house and then turn up here?"

"You're still in hospital then?"

"I hope to get out today. Don't change the subject."

"I was worried about you obviously."

"I'm fine. Now I am anyway. Why couldn't you have just waited until I got in touch with you?"

"But you didn't get in touch did you?"

"It was a couple of days Kirk for Christ's sake. You won't believe the shit you've caused me."

"Has your old man left you?" I said a little too optimistically.

"You think this is all a fucking joke don't you? You don't care one iota about how your actions affect other people."

"That's not true. I'm always thinking about ways I can upset the Chinese."

"See what I mean," snapped Lucy. "Nothing matters to you does it Kirk? You've completely fucked up my family with your stupid antics. Dave has gone mental."

"Mental? You mean he's like me now?"

"You know damn well what I mean. The kids are in bits. It's been bad enough with me being in hospital without all this shit on top."

"I wonder what you thought might happen when you climbed into the bed of a madman?"

"Well I certainly didn't expect this Kirk that's for sure."

"So it's okay to fuck up my life but not yours."

"How the hell have I fucked up your life?"

"You really haven't got a clue have you fat head?"

"That's because you're talking shit Kirk. Your life is one big fuck up, we both know that. And now you've managed to make mine one as well."

"You reckon?" I could feel my face going red. "I might have only got started. Did you ever think of that? Have you really got any idea what I am capable of? As you say, I'm mental and I have nothing else to lose."

"Don't threaten me Kirk. I can't cope." Her voice was cracking.

"All I did was love you fat head. I still love you. You knew exactly what kind of person I was when you got involved with me. I've never once hidden anything from you."

"I didn't think you'd do this. Just stay away Kirk. Please," she begged.

"I love you Lucy," I said and hung up.

I threw the phone on the sofa and went straight to the hallway mirror. I instantly started shouting 'cunt' at myself full blast. I could see a further change in the face looking back at me. The similarities to me were striking but I could clearly see that it wasn't my reflection.

"CUNT!" I continued to shout for a further hour. However, I suddenly stopped, pulled on some shoes and marched out of the house. I didn't even notice the shoes were an odd pair or that I had no socks on. I was off to the barber's on a mission and I wasn't bothered about such sartorial cock ups. My appearance had to change and the hair that I had groomed for so many years had to come off. All of it.

An hour later the elderly barber was brushing the loose hair away from the back of my neck and I was staring intently at the large mirror in front of me, admiring my new bald look. The face that looked back at me; the shaven head, the scary eyes, the drawn in cheeks, was looking less and less like I remembered myself to be. I eventually managed to pull myself away from the mirror long enough to pay the old man, who was now beginning to look like he wished he'd closed up early for the day. I paid him, not waiting for my change and stomped down the road to the Co-op. I was in desperate need of ham and lots of it. In fact the very thought of it was making me feel aggressive. I was definitely having one of my bad ham days. I'd had plenty of them before; mostly stress related and the only way to fix it was the quick consumption of large amounts of ham.

Once inside the supermarket I headed straight for the deli counter and took one of the tickets with numbers on it and waited impatiently to be told I was next. Fortunately The queue was small and number 43 was soon called.

"I need ham," I practically barked at a short tubby woman with a worrying squint of some sort.

"Certainly sir. What sort would you like?"

This immediately threw me so I replied, "pig ham and lots of it."

The shop assistant's face took on a nervous look. "I meant would you prefer smoked or unsmoked?"

"What kind of person do you take me for? Of course I don't want smoked." I pointed at some ham that had already been sliced. "Give me eighty slices of that stuff."

"Eighty slices?" The woman repeated.

"Okay make it twenty four. No, scrub that. I'll take two dozen."

After what seemed like an eternity I was finally sat on a bench outside the shop and cramming the ham into my mouth in an aggressive ham eating frenzy. An elderly chap with a greedy looking spaniel sat down beside me and I wasted no time in telling him about my ham needs.

"I fucking love ham," I said loudly. "Sometimes I get so angry when I haven't had any for a while that I go mental. Once I chopped down my neighbour's cherry tree. She refused to believe it was a ham related incident. Nor did my ex wife for that matter. Fucking heathens. I set fire to my mates shed last year. I hadn't had any ham in weeks. I told him not to get upset about it but he went ballistic. Stupid prick. The shed was falling apart anyway. His wife wanted to report me to the police for Christ's sake. What the hell is wrong with people?"

I turned to the old man but there was no sign of him or his dog. I looked up and down the street but he was gone. I thought about looking for him as I wanted him to know about my mates wife's threat of the police but just then my phone began to ring. I thought it may be Lucy calling to apologise but it was Craney.

"Wahay matey," he shouted down the phone. "What are you doing?"

"Aggressive ham eating. Two dozen slices of the thick cut stuff. I was feeling a bit violent."

"Ham related aggression eh?" Craney said non- plussed. *He* understood.

"Yeah, I've not been myself."

"Me neither," Craney replied. "We ought to hook up and form a community or something."

"Yeah, a leaning community or something."

Our conversation carried on in much the same vein before he said cryptically, "me and Andy are planning a special surprise for you."

"Go on," I said and waited.

"You'll see soon enough. Let's just say it's our very own contribution to the May Day CROUCH."

"You did the graffiti Craney," I said. "That was more than enough."

"Just look at this as a Craney special." With that he laughed and hung up. I couldn't begin to think what he had planned but no doubt it would be something ridiculous and probably illegal. I stared at my phone, wondering whether to ring Lucy but in the end decided against it and instead walked the short distance up the road to Peacocks. I was hoping to give Mr Jones a bit of abuse but he was nowhere to be seen. I cursed and headed home. When I got there Gemma greeted me with the words, "what the fuck have you done now?"

"It was a ham related decision," I answered predictably and then also predictably went to the hallway mirror.

"You look like you've just escaped from Auschwitz Kirk," Gemma said standing behind me and looking at my reflection over my shoulder.

"Good," I said just as the girls appeared. They both took one look at me and screamed. Gemma took a photo of me on her phone and sent it straight to Nikki.

"I can't get over how different you look mate. It's really spooky."

"I know. I am changing everyday."

"Listen, are you okay with me going over to my sister's tonight? She's doing my hair for me."

"Yeah I'm fine," I answered looking at her via the mirror.

"No funny stuff Kirk okay? Any problems you ring me."

I nodded. No funny stuff. I went back to concentrating on the mirror. The next thing I knew it was dark and I was laying face down on the kitchen floor.

CHAPTER TWENTY

HUMPTY DUMPTY FELL OFF THE WALL

CROUCHING Community Membership 9466

"What day is it?" I said to Annie who for some reason was in Gemma's kitchen. She was standing over me, her white hair standing out starkly in the darkness. She ignored my question and handed me a glass of water.

"Drink this," she said coolly passing it to me.

"Where's Gemma?" I asked but again received no answer, so I gulped the water down and laid back down, this time rolling onto my back. I stared up at Annie trying to make out her expression but it was too dark and I didn't have my glasses on. Instead I was greeted by an image of some pale angel peering down on me from high above. The one point of reference I had, the peroxide white hair, seemed to float unattached and gave off a ghostly impression. I felt cold even though I was sure I was perspiring. In fact my t-shirt was stuck to me with sweat. I shivered violently and Annie or whoever it was handed me a blanket or something which I gratefully grabbed. I considered getting up but something inside my head told me not to. I should stay exactly where I was. "Do I look normal?"

"That depends how you define normal Mr CROUCHER."

"Ah so it is you Annie. I can't really see you."

"I know Mr CROUCHER. You can't really see anything can you?"

She was right. The darkness enveloped her totally, the floating white image of her hair fading to nothing...

"You're a cunt!" I shouted again and again into the mirror at the bald man looking back at me.

"Kirk, shut the fuck up and get in here," Gemma called out from the kitchen.

I shouted a few more times at the stranger and went to find Gemma. She was stood looking out of the window, her back to me; a large glass of wine in her hand. Without turning she said, "I know you've stopped taking your medication. What the hell has gotten into you?"

"They stopped me getting a stiffy," I replied honestly.

"So it's been a while then?" Gemma turned now to face me. She didn't look impressed.

"What day is it Gem?"

"Don't change the fucking subject Kirk. Have you any idea how close you came last night to getting arrested? Or sectioned for that matter?"

I shook my head. "What the hell are you on about Gem?"

"Still in denial then?" Gemma said tersely raising her eyebrows.

"Gemma, I don't know what the hell you are going on about," I answered her truthfully.

"The worrying thing is Kirk, I believe you." Gemma reached for a glass and poured me a large slug of wine. She handed it to me and said, "*what do you* remember about last night?"

I thought for a minute, a nervous feeling coming over me. Obviously something had happened and as hard as I thought all I could recall is shouting in the mirror and waking up face down on the kitchen floor. "I remember Annie," I said suddenly, a vague image of her popping up somewhere at the back of my mind.

"Kirk, you threatened to burn Lucy's house down."

"What?" I said incredulously.

"You made Annie drive you to her house and apparently caused a right scene. Annie said you hammered on the front door and a man, who it turns out was Lucy's dad, answered the door. You started shouting a load of random shit and finished up telling him that if he didn't get Lucy out of bed you'd burn the house down."

"Is Lucy home?" I eagerly asked, which led Gemma to explode.

"Kirk, her husband came down here threatening to break your neck. I was half tempted to let him."

"Where was I?"

"Where do you think? Standing in front of the mirror shouting at yourself. I think it put him off a bit when he saw you. Poor Annie had to beg her parents not to call the police and that you were ill. It was one hell of a night."

I shook my head and said quietly, "I don't remember any of it."

"Mate you are unwell. I should have stepped in earlier. All this 'cunt' shouting and stuff. You have to start taking your pills again. In fact I insist on it. It's non negotiable."

I nodded sullenly, not quite able to take in what I was being told. The only thing that seemed to be registering was the fact that Lucy was out of hospital. Saying that, I had no idea if she actually was home or not. I really couldn't remember.

"And I'm taking that fucking mirror down in a minute," Gemma snapped, interrupting my thoughts. "Oh yeah, Annie will be here in a bit. She's a sweetheart, I tell you. She's been really worried about you. She must have rang me five times today already, checking if you've woken up. I'm taking the girls to the hairdresser's when she arrives; she can keep an eye on you. Just bloody behave yourself."

Annie was true to her word and half an hour later we had the house to ourselves. I listened intently but offered no opinion as Annie described the night's events. The scenes she described were as shocking as Gemma had said. I felt a sickening pain in the pit of my stomach as I was told about my crazy behaviour. Eventually it was too much for me and I rushed out of the sitting room only to find that Gemma had been true to her word and removed the mirror. For a few seconds I stood and stared at the wall not knowing what to do but then remembered the bathroom was full of mirrors. I shot up the stairs and immediately started shouting 'cunt' at myself the minute I reached the bathroom. A few seconds later Annie's reflection appeared in the mirror, a look a concern spread across her face.

I turned to face her and bellowed, "I'm the head of the CROUCHING community!" Then added quietly, "you are nothing." I turned back to the mirror and started shouting 'cunt' at the grinning face staring back at me. When the stranger began to laugh I punched the mirror with all my force causing it to shatter. One large piece remained attached to the wall and I pulled it off and held it up to look at. Annie had a look of shock on her face and was about to say something when I murmured, "this is what you've done to me," and stuck the shard of glass into my forehead. I pressed as hard as I could and then dragged it down as far as my eyebrow. Blood instantly gushed from the wound and I heard Annie let out a piercing scream. I dropped the piece of mirror and stood motionless as the blood poured down my face and onto my shirt.

"Oh my God Kirk," I heard Annie say more than once. "Oh my God."

"It was a ham related incident," I said looking at the blood now dripping all over Gemma's favourite cream fluffy towel which Annie had handed me.

"Right, press that against your head Kirk. Hard. We need to get you to A & E," Annie said quickly regaining her composure.

"Can't you sort it out? You're a doctor aren't you?"

"Kirk, listen to me. All I want you to do is press the towel hard against the wound. You need stitches. Quite a few by the look of it. Now come on." She pushed me out of the bathroom and guided me to her car. By the time we got to the hospital twenty minutes later I looked like I had been in a car crash such was the blood over me. Annie herself was also covered.

"What day is it?" I asked as she ushered me into the A & E department, but she ignored my question, instead went about speaking to a nurse. I wandered off aimlessly, ignoring the people in the waiting room who were as one, staring at me. A man holding his arm gingerly walked towards me with a young looking male nurse and I said, "wanking accident?" The nurse said something about sitting down but I had already walked by. I heard Annie shouting for me to go back to the reception desk but I ignored her. Eventually a nurse guided me into a small room which appeared like a mini operating theatre and an Indian doctor put twenty odd stitches in my forehead. I tried to listen to what Annie and an officious looking woman were talking about but it was impossible due to the Indian doctor's continuous chatter. Finally, after what seemed an eternity the doctor bandaged over the stitches and I was able to leave. Annie told me to sign some forms which she had filled in and two and a half hours after smashing the mirror I was back in the kitchen, once more being subjected to the wrath of Gemma. She was even more angry now about my self imposed pill ban and insisted on me taking my medication in front of her along with two suspicious looking pain killers the doctor had given to Annie. Whatever they were they knocked me out, no doubt combining with my own to make a potent cocktail.

I awoke on the sofa; the sun was shining in on me through the open blinds. I checked my watch. It said ten past ten. I must have slept all night. I immediately noticed the dull throbbing from my self inflicted wound. The throb rose to a real sharp pain once I sat up. I cursed and shouted to Gemma. There was no response but I could hear a clumping coming from above me and guessed she was upstairs making the beds or something. Thankfully there was a pint glass full of water on the small coffee table beside me and I drank almost the whole of it without coming up for air. I took a few minutes to get my thoughts together and made my way to the computer. I turned it on and immediately came face to face with a message asking for my password. This was new to me and I cursed loudly. I shouted for Gemma again but still got no reply. I decided a coffee would help so went to the kitchen to fill the kettle. I was surprised to see Gemma in there doing some ironing.

"Didn't you hear me calling you?"

"I guessed it was about the computer," she replied without looking up.

"Yeah what's going on with this password lark?"

"You are banned from it until further notice Kirk. Oh and your phone's also gone by the way."

I couldn't believe what I was hearing and let Gemma know. "What the fuck Gem? I've got the May Day CROUCH to sort out."

"No you don't. Annie's got everything in hand and I've spoken to Andy. You are under doctor's orders to rest." Gemma stopped ironing and finally looked at me.

"That's ridiculous. I'm the head of the CROUCHING community for God's sake. I have loads to do before Sunday. What day is it anyway?"

"You are going nowhere Kirk. In fact if you do, the only place you will end up is in hospital. In fact the only reason you were not sectioned yesterday was because Annie pulled some strings and her, me and Nikki agreed with your mental health nurse to ensure one of us is with you at all times and that you have no access to your phone or the computer." I was about to say something but Gemma raised a hand to silence me. "Kirk, you either do as you are told or I ring the quack. There is no debating it. In fact if you so much as hint at becoming psychotic or start coming out with crap I will have no qualms about sending you to hospital." She placed the iron on the kitchen worktop and walked around the ironing board coming up to stand in front of me. "Kirk, sweetheart," she said softly, "you have to listen to me. You need to rest. I can't have another day like yesterday." Tears welled in her eyes as she said this.

"Do you know if Lucy is home?" I asked as I hugged her. "I need to speak to her Gem."

"Mate, you are probably the last person on earth she wants to speak to at the moment."

"I need her Gem. I miss her." I did need her. None of this would have happened if Lucy hadn't left me hanging out to dry.

"I know mate. She'll get in touch when she's ready," Gemma said trying to reassure me but failing miserably.

I made us both a drink and we went out onto the decking. The sun was warm and we sat on the green plastic chairs that were scattered about haphazardly. Gemma said Annie was picking me up a new prescription of something or other and would be dropping it around later. I shrugged then asked, "tell me, do you think Annie is trying to take over the CROUCHING community?"

"Don't be ridiculous. She's a fucking wonder where you're concerned. I tell you this, if it wasn't for her you'd be locked up in a straight jacket by now."

I grunted, "she's up to something. It wouldn't surprise me if she had a sideways fucking fanny."

"You mean you haven't found out yet?" Gemma laughed. When I didn't answer her she turned to face me and said, "I've got something to cheer you up. Have a look at this." She played around with her phone then passed it to me.

"I thought you said no phones."

"Just look," she snapped.

I turned the phone away from the sun and looked at the screen. On it was a photo of Smeaton's Tower, the lighthouse on the Hoe; Plymouth's well loved sea front. Wrapped around the lighthouse in a sort of spiral going all the way from the viewing point at the top, down to the entrance gate at its foot, was a huge white banner of some sort. I could see huge black letters reading 'CROUCH' and 'May' from the angle the photo was taken.

"So this was what Craney was up to," I said laughing. "It's brilliant. God knows how they got away with it."

"Apparently a load of Andy's work crowd went up there in the early hours with ladders. It's been all over the local news. So you see Mr Christie, you really don't have to worry about your May Day CROUCH. Everyone's doing their bit."

I shook my head and asked her if there were any mirrors left in the house.

CHAPTER TWENTY ONE

SLEEPING WITH THE ENEMY

CROUCHING Community Membership   9,783

When I awoke I turned to see Nikki sat reading a magazine. I was in bed this time, so Gemma was good to her word about keeping me under orders. I felt absolutely drained and totally shattered. No doubt I was being administered the 'chemical cosh' to keep me sedated and this, added to days of not sleeping was knocking me senseless. I looked at the big shoe and fell back to sleep.

When I woke up again it was dark. My mouth was so dry I could barely move my tongue. I leant over to where I hoped a drink would be and thankfully my hand found a

glass. I gulped the water until the glass was empty and slumped back down onto the mattress. I became aware of a presence in the room and then suddenly realised someone was sleeping beside me. I turned over to see Annie's white hair sticking up from under the duvet. I fell back asleep.

Nikki shook me and handed me some pills and a glass of water. I swallowed them on auto pilot.

I woke up to find Gemma stood over me with a mug of coffee, a plate of sandwiches, a glass of water and more pills. "What day is it?" I asked but can't remember what she said.

It was dark again although the room was lit by Annie's laptop. She was sat cross legged on the bed in front of it frowning. I sat up and tried to focus. "I'm the fucking head..."

Nikki laughed as I almost fell over trying to stand upright. Eventually I made it to the bathroom to take a leak. I had to sit down and do it. I stared across at the small mirror opposite. Some weird looking bloke looked back at me. I didn't recognise him at all.

Gemma shook me. A woman I didn't recognise peered down at me. I think she asked me some questions.

I dreamt about climbing on top of a huge red shed.

I woke up and it was pitch black. I rolled over but Annie wasn't there. I fell back asleep.

Nikki said, "no, Lucy hasn't rang Kirk. Or sent a text. I checked your phone just now. Craney wanted to come round but I put him off for the minute. He told me to tell you that you're a gay prick. Annie's going to change your bandage tonight. Do you want some lunch?"

Annie told me to sit up and I struggled to lift my head. "Come on Mr CROUCHER, help me a bit." I said nothing as she removed the bandage from my head before gently cleaning the wound. I refused to make any comment about how much it hurt. Gemma came in with a coffee and a piece of fruit cake and looked closely at my head. The two girls said something but I didn't hear what it was. I think they were deciding whether to go out CROUCHING without me. "It's looking a bit healthier at last Mr CROUCHER," Annie said but I didn't believe her. I slept.

I woke up and it felt like I had been asleep for weeks. I could hear the hoover outside on the landing and music blaring over the top of its noise. I pulled myself out of bed and sat staring at the big shoe. I was cold with a damp sweat clinging to me and I didn't smell particularly great. I struggled to the bathroom, knocking into Gemma on the way. She seemed pleased to see me out of bed but still shouted at me to 'mind where I was fucking going.'

I quickly stripped and climbed into the bath. I switched on the shower, just remembering to pull the shower curtain across before the floor would have been flooded. The trouble was, by doing this I managed to get my bandage soaking wet. I cursed and let my head be drenched. The feeling of the warm water rushing over my face felt wonderful and I stood practically motionless for an eternity. In fact it was only when Gemma banged on the door and asked if I was still alive that I remembered to reach for some shower gel. I washed quickly and thoroughly, unsure when I would next get the chance. Eventually I gingerly removed the wet bandage and turned nervously to the small mirror. Even I was shocked to see the horror show face that stared back at me. I looked so gaunt and pale I could have just done a year in solitary confinement. My eyes no longer sparkled, but were sunken back into my skull, the left one looking scarily stretched open by the lowest of the stitches pulling the eyelid upwards. The wound itself looked incredible. Worryingly so. Along with my shaven head the wound made me look completely different.

"Now I am you," I said to my reflection. "We are the same person." We looked truly awful...

When I had dressed and brushed my teeth I went downstairs to be greeted by Gemma who handed me a mug of coffee. For a moment neither of us said anything. In the end it was me who who broke the silence.

"I'm really sorry Gem," I said and could feel tears welling up in my eyes.

"Let's just put it all down to a bad ham related incident shall we?" Gemma replied and threw her arms around me. We hugged for a long time. I guessed that Gemma also had tears but didn't want to show me them. Finally she released me and said, "right you fucking nuisance, can I get back to some sort of normality now?" I nodded and for the next hour Gemma brought me up to date on what she knew of the May Day CROUCH news. Then she gave me my pills and I fell asleep.

"You snore like a pig Mr CROUCHER," said Annie who was sitting up in the bed beside me reading.

"What?" I said still half asleep.

"Gemma said you are back with us.

"Did she?"

"I've never met anyone sleep as much as you have."

"What day is it?"

"Is that all you ever say?"

"No one ever tells me." I could sense Annie wasn't happy.

"Why have you removed your bandage?" She asked.

"I knew you weren't happy."

"You're right, I'm not over impressed with you at the moment but not because of the bandage. I expected you to do that to be honest." She turned to look at me. "Do you remember all the things you said to me?"

"About ham?"

"No Mr CROUCHER, not ham. About me trying to kill you and take over the CROUCHING community? About me trying to poison your dogs? About me digging holes in the back garden? About me wanking off Craney in the Spar shop on North Hill? Shall I go on?"

"Did he enjoy it?"

"I'm glad you think it's funny. Do you know at one point you even told a nurse that I had, and I quote, 'fingered myself in front of your elderly parents.'

I tried not to grin but I couldn't help myself. "I wasn't in control of my mind. I cannot be held responsible for my words or actions."

"Well you owe me big time. Not to mention having to bloody nurse you."

"Have you been looking at my penis whilst I slept?"

"Yes and it's tiny."

I let out a grunt then asked, "so how's the May Day CROUCH shaping up?"

"Very well indeed; everything is under control and your community awaits you. Oh and the Smeaton's Tower thing Craney and his lot did was amazing. It's even been on the tele. And my student buddies have been doing loads. They went to..."

I fell back to sleep.

Gemma woke me up pulling back the curtains. For some reason I instantly said, "you've talked to her haven't you?"

"You made me jump mate."

"You have though haven't you?"

"What the fuck are you on about now?"

"Lucy of course. You've spoken to her."

Gemma came over to me and sat down on the bed. "I suppose you're well enough to know now," she sighed. "Yes we talked."

"Well, what did she say?"

"I told her how poorly you had been."

"And what did she say to that?"

"She's scared mate. Afraid of what you're capable of. You're lucky that she managed to persuade her family not to go to the police. I explained what we'd all been going through here with you. To be honest I don't think she understood how ill you are. She said she always found your condition funny."

"Yeah It's really fucking funny," I said, shaking my head.

"You have to understand that people don't get to see the other side of it like me and Nikki do."

"But I love her Gem."

"Well mate you are going to have to stop loving her because I can't see her family letting you get within ten miles of her." She got up from the bed. "By the way am I safe bringing the girls home from my sister's now?"

I felt totally embarrassed. "Yeah, it will be good to have them home. I feel really bad about it."

Gemma laughed. "Are you kidding me? Its been fucking great."

An hour later I finally had the house to myself for the first time in what felt like years. I was showered and dressed and hovering over the home telephone. I swear I could actually feel my stomach turn. I picked up the receiver and dialled Lucy's number. I listened to it ring and then go to voicemail. "Fat head, it's me. I am back in the land of the living. Meet me up the Josh at midday today. I need to speak to you. Don't back out as I'll only come around your house and I'm sure you don't want that. See you soon."

I grabbed a jacket and left the house. The head of the CROUCHING community was back.

CHAPTER TWENTY TWO

LUCY IN THE SKY WITH DIAMONDS

CROUCHING Community Membership 9,999

I walked slowly but purposefully through the damp streets, noticing that I got more than a few strange looks from people I passed. I boomed a loud 'good morning' to a woman waiting at a bus stop and she looked petrified. I missed the sausage kings on a day like this. I could have told them all my troubles. It dawned on me how much I had lost in the last few weeks. I couldn't lose Lucy. I had to have her in my life. I knew that this would be my one and only chance to salvage anything of our relationship and that thought was enough to make me stop and do a bit of 'leaning.' I found a nice lamp post of the old wooden variety and spent five minutes leaning against at a number of angles. I considered a quick CROUCH outside a particularly attractive pillar box set into an old wall opposite St Mary's church but decided at the last minute to forgo the temptation. I had to keep focused.

The pub was empty bar an old chap in the corner reading a newspaper. I ordered a bottle of Pils and considered the last month or so. It had been a vintage 'episode' even by my standards. Yet I had somehow managed to come out the other side. I knew I was lucky. The fallout had been and no doubt would continue to be, profound and affect many people and as usual it was those closest to me who got the worst of it. This time I had reached the very limits and was lucky to have made it back down to earth. There had been times when I had felt like a lost soul floating around the very edge of the universe. Now I was back and by recent standards, reasonably healthy.

I had just ordered a second bottle of lager when I became aware of Lucy's presence. I smelt her before I saw her. I turned around and there she was. Lucy. She looked fantastic. A half second glance was all it took for me to know how much I longed for her. She was dressed in tight blue jeans with her customary very high heeled shoes and a smart red leather coat. Her expression was one of absolute shock when she took in my new look. She even took a step back unconsciously.

"Thanks for coming," I said nervously, unsure of how she'd react.

"I didn't have much choice did I?" Lucy answered trying not to stare at my forehead.

"I wouldn't have gone to your house Lucy. I just wanted to get you here."

"Yeah right," she said shaking her head.

I ignored her response and ordered her a vodka and coke, guessing she would need one. Neither of us said another word until we were sat at a corner booth. It seemed years since she had sexily swallowed the wafer thin ham here, yet it was mere weeks. So much had happened since that glorious night.

"I was going to bring the big shoe for you. You know, like a peace offering."

"I didn't come here to listen to you go on about that fucking shoe Kirk," said Lucy coldly. "I hope you haven't forced me up here just to talk shit."

This was not the way I had planned to open my make or break plea to her. "I'm sorry fat head," I apologised. "I'm nervous. You make me nervous."

Lucy threw back her head as if she was about to laugh but didn't. "I make *you* nervous?

That's a good one. Kirk, every time the phone rings or there is a knock at the door I have a heart attack. Have you any idea how much shit you've caused me?"

I looked at her with a blank expression, offering nothing.

"You really don't give a flying fuck do you?"

"I've been having a hard time Lucy," I said and was about to go on but Lucy cut me short.

"Kirk, don't give me all the mental crap. I've had a real illness as you well know and the last thing I needed was for you to cause so much hassle for me."

I looked down at my bottle of Pils. I couldn't bring myself to look at her. "I'm sorry," I mumbled.

For a full minute neither of us said a word. It was me who finally broke the silence. Still looking down I said, "listen to me Lucy, I love you. I'm crazy about you. I fucked up, I know. I always fuck up. It's in my nature. Everything that's ever any good in my life I fuck up. The minute we met I knew deep down I'd end up fucking it up." Lucy went to say something but I raised a hand to stop her. "Let me finish, there's stuff I need to say." I removed my glasses in an attempt to be more sincere but probably just looked more disturbing than ever. "I know I've been an idiot. Half the stuff that's happened I don't even remember doing but if you say I did it I believe you. It seems I've pissed off just about everyone that matters to me in the last few weeks. You mock my illness Lucy but by now you ought to have a pretty good idea how serious it is. I know you've been ill and how poorly you've been but don't ever think that just because my illness is of the mind and not the body that I'm any more healthy that you." I banged my hand down on the table and added, "look at me Lucy. Do I look a well man to you?" I stared at her in an attempt to emphasize my point. "When you went abroad I suffered a pretty bad manic episode. I'm not talking just lying face down on the kitchen floor, I mean hallucinations. Or being laid across a railway track tying to kill myself. And slicing my head open because I thought it was someone else's. I mean wandering the streets like a zombie for nights on end. I mean staring in a mirror for hours and fucking hours and looking at the bogeyman staring back.

Yes you have been un well Lucy but you will recover. I never will." Tears had welled up in Lucy's eyes. I reached across the table and placed my hand on hers. "People laugh at me. I make people laugh. People are attracted to me because of my crazy antics and ridiculous ideas. They don't have a clue. To them it's all a joke but to me it's my life. My life," I said again to emphasise the point. I stopped to take a swig from my bottle. My eyes never left Lucy's. "I don't CROUCH because I *want to* CROUCH. I do it because I *have to*. Just as I *have to* hunt midgets and *I have* to lay face down on the kitchen floor and I *have to* hide in hedges making animal noises. I don't have a choice in the matter. I thought you of all people would realise that Lucy. I thought we understood each other. You once said that nothing I did would upset or offend you. And yet the very first time you come face to face with the madness in me you run a mile. You realise that perhaps you don't like me so much after all. You're a hypocrite Lucy. It's like falling in love with someone with cancer then dumping them when their hair falls out."

I finally let her speak. "It's nothing like that Kirk and you know it. You came to my home. You caused a real shit storm. My kids are in fucking bits Kirk. I cannot have that."

"You caused that when you decided to climb into my bed. Were you thinking about your kids when I had my cock up your arse?"

"Stop it Kirk," Lucy snapped and withdrew her hand from mine. I was surprised she hadn't done it sooner. "My children have to come first. I didn't expect you to go into some sort of mental meltdown just because I'd gone away for a few days. If I did I would never had let things get so complicated with you."

"Sex on your terms," I said tasting acid.

"You know what I mean."

"Do I Lucy? All I know is that you came into my life, a beautiful bonanza from the Gods. Summer had come early and then you left so quickly you didn't even turn the lights off. The fact is I'm still in the light Lucy; your light. Come back in Lucy, the lights are still on." I didn't know whether to be impressed by this line or to cringe.

Tears were now rolling down Lucy's face. "I can't Kirk, you know I can't."

"You can fat head. I know you love me still."

"Don't Kirk," Lucy pleaded. "Please don't. I can't deal with this at the moment. There's just too much stuff that's happened. And my children need me more than ever. They've only just stopped thinking that their mum is going to die at any moment."

I leaned across the table and this time grabbed hold of both hands. "Tell me you don't love me."

"Stop it Kirk, that's unfair."

"I need you in my life Lucy," I pleaded. "I really need you."

Now the tears were really flowing. Lucy made no attempt to wipe them away. "If only you hadn't ruined everything. Why couldn't you have just let things run their course instead of jumping in with both feet?"

"I thought I'd just explained that?"

"I just can't take the risk Kirk," Lucy said finally wiping at the tears. "I just can't. I never expected all this."

I said nothing for a moment. I just looked at her and for the first time saw the look of absolute dejection on her face. I watched her age before my eyes. It dawned on me that she was trapped. The chance I had offered I had dashed away from under her and now she was right back to square one. In fact she was now way worse off than she ever was. For Lucy life would now be unbearable. She looked sad.

"I won't lose you," I said again.

"Are you not listening Kirk? I can't do this anymore. I won't do it anymore."

"Lucy," I said her name hoping it would help. "I'm fine now. My crazy period is over. I'm good old Kirk again."

She smiled at me weakly, her already pale face now almost translucent. "The damage is done and it can't be fixed. Not by you anyway. You are right; I do still have feelings for you. Of course I do. Although I can't say I'm over enthused about your new look." She smiled sadly at me again. "But like I said, I have to put my children first."

"Listen," I said almost conspiratorially. "I get it. I really do. Take as long as you need sweetheart. I'm not going anywhere. I'm not going to lose you."

"No you listen Kirk. It's over. It has to be. You have to listen to me. I need you to understand."

I looked at the love of my life sat across the table; so close I could lean forward and kiss her, yet so distant I may as well be a hundred miles away from her. I could see in her eyes that she had made up her mind. The decision was final. I could see the pain too. Yes she loved me but it wasn't enough. Sometimes love doesn't conquer all. I felt my body, which I had summoned to rise from days of slumber, begin to sag. It was like a giant hand had pressed down on me and pushed me down into the seat. I was visibly shrinking in front of her.

"Kirk, are you listening to me? It's over. I'm really sorry. I still care about you and no doubt will worry about you and of course I will miss you, but it's over. I need you to understand. Please don't make this a problem. I can't live my life worrying from one day to the next if you are going to turn up on my doorstep or do something stupid." Her eyes pleaded with me.

I looked away from her and stared at the pool table. Then my head dropped. The battle was lost. I had nothing left. It was over. We sat in silence for what felt an eternity. Eventually I heard Lucy's chair move and felt her cold hand touch my face. She let out a sigh and said softly, "you're a very special person Kirkland Christie." She kissed me gently on the cheek and walked away.

"Yeah, special fucking needs!" I shouted after her but she had already gone.

For a while I didn't move. I focused on the pattern in the carpet as if it might somehow contain a mystical answer to my problems amongst the whirls. When I couldn't find one I stood up and drained the last of my drink. I wandered out of the pub and onto the busy street outside, almost bumping into people as I half staggered along the pavement. As if drawn by an invisible magnet I found myself stood outside Peacocks, staring blankly in through the window. The shop was quiet and there was no sign of Mr Jones so I turned away and walked out into the road and laid down on the wet tarmac and stared up at the grey sky. "I'm Dick Van Dyke," I said quietly to myself and closed my eyes.

I felt like I was lying there for hours but it was probably a matter of seconds before concerned voices began to fill the air. I felt a hand touch my arm and shouted, "don't touch me," at the top of my voice. I heard more voices and even my name being called. I repeated my warning not to touch me before screaming, "I'm Dick Van Dyke," over and over. Someone said 'Chitty Chitty Bang Bang' and I finally opened my eyes. A sea of worried looking faces looked down at me. I shouted, "don't touch me" again and closed my eyes.

"He says he's Dick Van Dyke," I heard a woman say loudly and then a man's voice saying something about me 'being the mad bloke who does the CROUCHING.' Then I heard a familiar voice in my ear. "Kirk sweetie. Can you hear me?"

I opened my eyes to see Sarah, a member of the community who had known me since my school days. "I'm Dick Van Dyke for God's sake," I said and saw her mouth the word 'ambulance' to someone I couldn't see. A man I vaguely recognised put a coat over me but I threw it off and shouted, "I don't feel the cold! I'm Dick Van Fucking Dyke!" I closed my eyes again, smiled to myself and waited for the men in the white coats to come and get me. Dick Van Dyke was leaving the stage.

CHAPTER TWENTY THREE

IS THIS A PIECE OF YOUR BRAIN?

CROUCHING Community Membership   10,458

The man who stood in the middle of the room thinking he was a tree for hours on end sat down next to me. He immediately began to make strange clucking noises from somewhere at the back of his throat. I turned and looked at him but said nothing. I had barely said half a dozen words in days. I say days but it could be weeks. I couldn't seem to get to grip with time now that my watch had been removed.

"The oak stands strong against all the evil in the world you know," the tree man said matter of factly. He liked a good oak tree. "But the yew grows old and wise."

I watched a nurse walk past carrying a box of crayons and felt tips. It must be almost lunch time. The morning's art class must be finished. Art was one of the many therapy classes that went on each day. One of the nurses had persuaded me to have a go but all I managed to do was draw a three legged dog with no tail.

"She has the look of the cedar," the tree man said loudly as he watched the nurse putting the art stuff away. "Or a lime in winter." He got back up and took a new pose. From what he had said the other day I think it was a sycamore tree. The nurse smiled at me as she walked back to the reception area but all I managed back was an involuntary twitch; a side affect of whatever strong drugs I was being pumped with.

"Almost lunchtime gentleman," the nurse called over her shoulder. "Roast beef today."

Niether of us answered her. I noticed that the tree man actively stared down at his feet when she spoke. I just stared blankly at her back and thought that I felt hungry now she had mentioned food. A couple of fat old ladies shuffled past, heading for the canteen. They gave the tree man a wide berth not that he noticed. He was now staring up at the ceiling. I found myself fixated on the ulcer like growths on one of the women's fat ankles. I had noticed them earlier this morning and they bothered me. I twitched again and this seemed to break the spell.

"Come on Mr Van Dyke. Time to feed the roots."

I followed the tree man into the small canteen robotically, picking up a tray and joining the queue of seven people. I counted them slowly. I was doing a lot of counting lately. When I reached the servery hatch I just nodded in response to each question and took my laden tray to a table where two youngish men were sat in silence. None of us offered a word throughout the whole meal. I ate robotically, clearing my plate but finding no enjoyment from the food. I took my plate back to the hatch as we had been told to do and poured myself a coffee. Taking a couple of digestives I wandered into the lounge where there was a number of comfy sitting chairs placed around a large flat screen television which was always on whether anyone was watching it or not. I sat down in front of it and stared blankly at the screen. A woman was saying something about a war somewhere. I paid no interest in what she was saying but enjoyed seeing the bombs exploding. I dunked a biscuit in the coffee, leaving a sizeable chunk floating in the mug. I stared sullenly at it then looked up at the TV again. A large group of people were doing a sort of squat and a young punk was saying something about a man getting well. It must have been a cancer charity thing or something. I dunked my other biscuit making sure I was extra careful not to lose it this time. When I looked at the screen again the weather forecast was on. Apparently summer was on the way.

THE END